L 45627

Medicine Walk
Reconnecting to Mother Earth

LAURIE LACEY

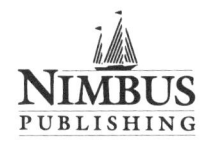

NIMBUS
PUBLISHING

This book is dedicated to my friends, and to everyone who loves and appreciates Mother Earth.

Copyright © 1999, Laurie Lacey

The author does not take responsibility for the misuse of information given in this book. Individuals seeking relief from serious illness should consult a qualified health practitioner. This book is not intended to replace the services of a health professional. Persons with serious psychological difficulties should consult a qualified psychologist or psychiatrist, and use this book under the direction of a professional.

All rights reserved. No part of this book may be reproduced, stored in a retrieval system or transmitted in any form or by any means without the prior written permission from the publisher, or, in the case of photocopying or other reprographic copying, permission from CANCOPY (Canadian Copyright Licensing Agency), 1 Yonge Street, Suite 1900, Toronto, Ontario M5E 1E5.

Nimbus Publishing Limited
PO Box 9301, Station A, Halifax, NS B3K 5N5
(902) 455-4286

Design: Joan Sinclair
Cover photo: Irwin Barrett
Illustrations by Laurie Lacey

Canadian Cataloguing in Publication Data
Lacey, Laurie.
Medicine walk
Includes index.
ISBN 1-55109-306-5
1. Medicinal plants.   2. Nature, Healing power of.   I. Title.
QK99.A1L33 1999   581.6'34   C99-950067-8

Nimbus Publishing acknowledges the financial support of the Canada Council and the Department of Canadian Heritage.

AUTHOR'S ACKNOWLEDGEMENTS

I wish to acknowledge and express my deep gratitude to all those people who, during the past couple of years, have encouraged my interest in exploring nature and the outdoor environment for therapeutic purposes. Thanks also to Judy and the staff at Arby's Restaurant, Bridgewater, Nova Scotia, where I wrote most of the initital draft for this book while sipping a cup of tea or coffe. Finally, my humble gratitude to the Spirit in my heart for the many ways it has found to inspire me over the years.

TABLE OF CONTENTS

Introduction   iv

CHAPTER 1   *Dismiss Fear: Affirm Joy and Happiness*   *1*
CHAPTER 2   *The Discovery of Special Places*   *10*
CHAPTER 3   *Using Our Special Places*   *19*
CHAPTER 4   *Coping with Stress the Natural Way*   *31*
CHAPTER 5   *Expanding Our Horizons*   *42*
CHAPTER 6   *Exploring Meditation*   *53*
CHAPTER 7   *Discovering the Wild Edibles*   *63*
CHAPTER 8   *Medicine Walk*   *77*
CHAPTER 9   *The Spirituality of Plants*   *98*

Medicinal Plant/Tree Index   *126*
with illustrations and preparation instructions
Food Plant/Tree Index   *133*
Plant/Tree Spirit Energy Index   *134*
Bibliography   *136*

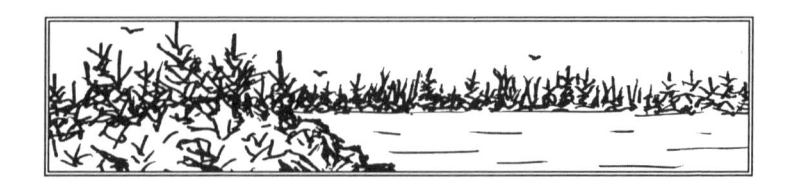

INTRODUCTION

> *I went to the woods because I wished
> to live deliberately; to confront only
> the essential facts of life, and see
> if I could not learn what it had to teach...*
>   Henry D. Thoreau
>   *Walden* in Krutch (ed.)
>   *Thoreau: Walden and Other Writings,* p. 172

THE world of nature is a source of inspiration, enjoyment, and peace in my life—a place of refuge and comfort during difficult periods or stressful situations, whenever they arise. Many people find refuge in a church or other edifice built by human hands or, when problems arise, they seek professional guidance. This is understandable. But my refuge is the forest; my altar, a large rock or a clump of witch hazel; my inspiration, the grandeur of a lake or, like the ancient Druids, an oak tree. My counsellor at one moment is a breeze whispering through pine needles; the next it is a spectacular sunset or the call of a distant crow. Such impressions help to create an intimate connection between our lives and the natural world. They can have a healing influence, affecting the innermost parts of our being.

  This book is the culmination of a life of outdoor experiences, and their translation into words that attempt to express the wonderful therapeutic value of the natural environment. However, the writing of this book was not easily accomplished; it occurred over a three-year period. The original manuscript was created as a self-published course in nature therapy.* Gradually it altered and expanded into its present form, not unlike an oak tree that matures slowly from an acorn into a beautiful tree.

II

I GREW up in a rural environment, spending much of my time in the forest and fields of the local neighbourhood. Looking back, I realize the beneficial role the natural world played in my life, especially during the early teen years. This was a time of personal turmoil for me, as it is for many teenagers. I worried a lot and suffered from anxiety. The anxiety largely resulted from a physical handicap that made me very shy and self-conscious. It was compounded by a profound hatred of school. The teachers offered little encouragement; in fact, several were downright nasty and, in hindsight, were probably unfit for their profession. It seemed to me that not one of them came even remotely close to understanding my situation. I rebelled against everything pertaining to the education system.

I quit grade seven two years in a row, once attending school for only 28 days of the term. I would purposely skip school by running away and hiding in the forest. I was not an ideal student. Often, I would climb a tree and remain hidden there until I missed the bus. The forest offered solace and a

---

* The title of this course is Nature Therapy for Health and Well-Being, and is available through the author.

means of escape from public education. I believe this was the first time that I applied nature therapy to personal problems.

A year later, I used the outdoor environment as a regular classroom. This wonderful experience happened because of the common-sense approach of my brother, Glenn, a school teacher himself. As a last resort to ensure I received a standard education, he enrolled me in a correspondence course so that I could continue learning at home, which I was successful in doing from grades seven through ten. Often, when the weather was good, I would do my work in the peaceful setting of the forest. Whenever he had free time, Glenn supervised my study, tutoring me in English, mathematics, and other subjects. I have fond memories of learning algebra under the nurturing influence of an old hemlock. I benefited immensely from that experience.

III

THERE are many benefits to the use of this book. It includes notes and exercises that may be used as aids to control stress, overcome fear, increase prosperity, and foster the ability to concentrate and meditate. I sincerely hope that this book will open avenues of self-discovery, teaching the reader to use the wonderful surroundings of the natural world for their therapeutic value; to experience the healing blessings of mother nature and the lessons she teaches.

One way to benefit from nature's gifts is to locate "special places," which are important for relating to the natural world and for establishing a feeling of connectedness to the earth. Locating your special places takes careful consideration. Don't rush the process simply for the sake of expediency, or because you are in a hurry to begin the exercises suggested. Choose locations that are quiet, peaceful, comfortable, safe, private, and accessible on a regular basis. It is important to have a place where you can appreciate nature under the most favourable conditions. It is useful to practise the exercises in sequence, noting those most effective for you, so you will have a core of exercises especially beneficial to your personal situation and circumstances.

In addition, I believe there is psychological and social value to the frequent use of affirmations in daily life. The use of affirmations is discussed at several points in this book, particularly in my discussion of the "transformation affirmation," which should be practised daily.

IV

This book offers a wide variety of exercises, many of which are given to expand the reader's appreciation of the natural world, and to deepen his or her awareness of the rich sensory impressions that nature provides. A number of the exercises have practical applications relating to problems such as poor concentration, fear, stress, or the failure to reach goals. A person may discover that a particular exercise on concentration, for example, will also be beneficial in relieving stress. The exercise may be the medicine we need at a particular moment in time. If so, treasure it and use it on a regular basis. Of course, these exercises are not magical solutions by themselves; however, used in conjunction with a positive attitude, they will prove quite beneficial.

The chapter on exploring the spiritual nature of plants was written to challenge the creative imagination of readers. There is much more behind physical reality than meets the eye, so to speak. We are conditioned by our culture to view and interpret sensory information in a certain way. But, if we are willing to entertain new ideas and possibilities, it is possible to break free from that conditioning. I ask you to do this as you read and contemplate my comments on the spirituality of plants.

I have tried to take into consideration how physically and/or mentally challenged individuals might approach the outdoor exercises and activities suggested here. While I realize that each person is unique, I have tried to make suggestions that are general enough to include most people, regardless of their circumstances. A person who is unable to fully participate in an exercise because of a disability, should do it to the best of his or her ability. No one should be excluded from experiencing the benefits of the natural world. This is a primary concern to me. It is easy to isolate people with acute disabilities from the natural landscape, either because we are overprotective or because we don't make the effort required to involve the disabled in nature-based activities. I applaud all those individuals and organizations who sponsor outdoor activities such as summer camps and other recreational events for the disabled.

It is my hope that after reading this book you will begin to explore the landscape on a regular basis; learn to identify the birds, animals, fishes, rocks, trees, and plant life in your environment. Make an effort to visit a new location every month, and hike favourite places often. Above all, let love and appreciation be your guide, so that you practise a kind, loving ethic in your everyday interaction with the wonderful environment around us.

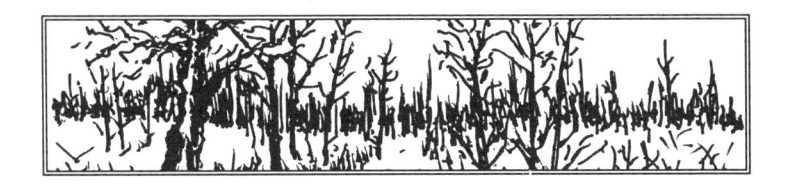

Chapter 1

DISMISS FEAR
Affirm Joy and Happiness

MANY people who spend time in the outdoors hiking and exploring have found themselves lost at least once in their lives. They know the feeling it engenders: a sinking feeling of anxiety—even panic—and a sense of urgency. Mind you, I haven't analysed my mental state when I've been lost, since I'm always too busy trying to figure out where I am in relation to the nearest point of familiarity in the landscape! But I can remember experiencing a lot of anxiety whenever I was lost during my teen years. I used to go hunting and occasionally find myself in the middle of a swamp or bog, wondering which way was home.

One autumn evening, several years ago, I got lost while walking in a forest that should have been familiar to me—instead, I quickly became disoriented. I found myself thinking the usual kinds of negative thoughts associated with the prospect of spending a night in the woods without equipment or supplies of any kind. I soon realized my situation wasn't so bad, and that I could at least start a fire if necessary. Thinking over the situation, I concluded there were two things in my favour: I knew there was a lake to the west of my location with which I was familiar, and I could easily ascertain its direction from the faint glow of the setting sun.

The walking was easy as I made my way around and over rotting tree branches, through a thick covering of leaves, and down a steep slope in the direction of the lake. To the east, I heard the deep sound of a raven croaking, as if it recognized my presence. A thick floor of leaves, which had fallen recently, made rustling sounds under my feet, while ahead of me was the faint glow of a "sundog." I recalled the many occasions when my father had spoken about sundogs. When one was to the west, he would say, "It's a sign of fair weather." A sundog to the south was a sign of rain. Often sundogs appear simultaneously, to the south and the west. When this happened, my father would watch the sky and note which sundog remained the longest. For instance, if a sundog to the south remained the longest, he would predict rain. In her book, *Folklore of Lunenburg County*, Helen Creighton writes that a sundog in the evening is a sign of rain. My father would have replied that this was so only if the sundog were in the south.

I was still considering the significance of the sundog phenomenon when I saw the water sparkling in the distance through a break in the tightly woven spruce branches in my immediate path. Struggling through the thick spruce I caught sight of the shoreline and realized that my position was a hundred metres or so south of where I had thought I was. It was difficult to believe that I had become lost in this area, although I have heard similar stories of it happening to people in familiar terrain. Perhaps the forest takes on a different appearance at certain periods of the day, changing its mood and altering itself. I considered this possibility and decided that the direction I travelled probably contributed to my predicament. The direction one travels is always important, as familiar things may take on a different appearance if approached from a different direction. I was travelling east; perhaps that was what confused me. I had always travelled west over that country. Many hikers, including myself, have noticed how the landscape can play games with one—how, for example, returning from a hike over the same ground one walked earlier gives an entirely new perception of the place.

It is easy to focus on the negative aspects of being lost, rather than considering it a positive learning experience. In my case, I was fortunate enough to be in an area that was normally familiar to me. A person is more likely to experience fear if lost in unfamiliar terrain. Under those circumstances it is normal to feel uncertainty and anxiety. Yet, even in this situation, it is very helpful to assume a positive and courageous approach to the problem.

II

NEGATIVE attitudes are common in society; they are present in most people. Indeed, negativity forms part of the ethos or nature of modern Western culture and society. Several years ago I became acutely aware of the extent of my own negativity. It was shocking, really. I was reading a popular self-help book in which the author discussed negative thought, especially self-criticism and the skeptical feedback we deal ourselves on a daily basis. He wrote about the pessimism we encounter in our friends, in the population in general, and in the media. He challenged his readers to note the number of times they gave themselves negative feedback of any kind in the run of an ordinary day. The next day I accepted the challenge. I was amazed! The day had hardly begun and I was counting in double-digits. The exercise was very revealing and marked the beginning of a readjustment in my thinking patterns. I realized the extent to which my thought processes proceeded in a manner detrimental to my own best interests. After all, if we wish to accomplish certain things with our lives, and to live in happiness and joy, the last thing we need is a negative attitude or a stream of negative thoughts moving through our consciousness.

As individuals interested in the outdoor experience, we can take steps to counter the tendency to view the world through negative glasses. We can engage the landscape in a creative dialogue, forging a new relationship between ourselves and the environment. We can choose to take part in nature-based activities that are a tonic to body, mind, soul, and spirit, and in this manner use our environment in a way that affirms a positive lifestyle. This affirmative commitment to things positive will inspire others and create health, enthusiasm, and joy in our lives.

I have meditated on a commitment to joyfulness while walking the shoreline of Minamkeak Lake at sunset, allowing the rays of the evening sun to bathe my face. In this way, I have used the sun as a stimulus to finding joy. Often my body responds, and I feel a tickling sensation of joy spreading outward from the pit of my stomach. I have also walked in the forest with this commitment singing in my head, and strolled along city streets with this joy uppermost in my thoughts. Anyone can make the decision to commit themselves to this philosophy—to affirm "joy" frequently, wherever they are and in whatever they are doing. It is my belief that this commitment creates a force much like magnetism, attracting people, places, and experiences of a pleasant, joyful nature.

Consider this example of the power of nature to stimulate a cleansing, healing experience. Several years ago I was hiking through a tall spruce forest when I found myself in a clearing with a large rock out-cropping overlooking flat marshland extending to the horizon. It rippled through the marsh, like waves over the surface of a lake. A gentle breeze caressed my face. As I stood there, my mind emptied—I could virtually feel the wind blowing through it, as if it were a house with all the windows and doors open. I was devoid of worry or concern of any kind. I realized the precious nature of the experience, and wondered how often we allow such healing moments to slip through our lives without notice, focussing instead on the so-called "big events" that bring headache and worry. As I walked home that day, I determined to pay attention to those experiences in the future, and to create the circumstances necessary for their occurrence.

Exercise 1: *The Power of Affirmations*

Go for a walk in the forest, along a beach, a place with a breathtaking view, or some other location that is both inspiring and invigorating. Relax. Take several minutes to examine in detail the beauty of your environment. Concentrate for a few moments on your body; feel the consciousness in each part of the body as you focus your attention. Slowly repeat this affirmation: *I am a positive, dynamic person. I think joyful thoughts. I feel joy at the present moment. This joy is in my consciousness and my body. I am a creative, joyful, loving person. My life is overflowing with abundant good.*

To be most effective, this affirmation should be repeated on a daily basis. In fact, if possible, repeat it several times daily. Upon rising in the morning, look in the mirror, give yourself a greeting smile and say the affirmation. Repeat it again at lunchtime or before beginning your afternoon schedule. Say the affirmation before retiring at night. As mentioned above, it is useful to use the affirmation in an outdoor setting, because the power behind your affirmation is the power behind, and in nature herself. Repeating the affirmation in a beautiful forest environment will serve as a reminder of this principle.

Several years ago I used affirmations on a regular basis for a time. I would drive to a special place in the country, park my car, and walk through the woods to a large boulder. Climbing the boulder, I would stand with arms outstretched, slowly repeating the words while anticipating much happiness in my life. Of course, saying an affirmation involves more than mechanically repeating the words—that isn't good enough! Philosophers such as Nicholas Roerich, Rudolph Steiner, Helen Blavatsky, Paracelsus, and others, believed that there is a tremendous amount of creative potential within the spoken word when said with feeling, sincerity, and understanding. You must think deeply on the affirmation, speaking each word with confidence and conviction. Always say your affirmation in a slow, deliberate fashion, concentrating on the words. Make the time for this practice daily. It will be time well spent.

As you repeat the affirmation, surrounded by the beauty and strength of nature, try to sense the power behind your words. Don't struggle to put power into your words. Know that the force of nature is already working for you. Know with the conviction of a magician or the faith of a saint that your affirmation is working to bring good into your life.

III

WHENEVER we doubt, worry, or fear that something isn't possible, we place an obstacle in our path, limiting the creative potential of the mind. That is why it is important to conquer our tendency to fear things unnecessarily. The natural world offers many opportunities in this regard. On a basic level, we may fear small things, such as the first time we venture out in a canoe or a kayak. Or, especially in spring, we may fear encountering a hungry bear in the woods, even though the likelihood of such an encounter is remote. Yet, if we succumb to such fears, we may never experience the delights of canoeing or walking the forest in the spring.

Fear is always a difficult foe, whether it is the fear of failure, of making changes in our lives, or of doing things that alter the status quo, even slightly. Even after we have overcome our fear of certain things, we shouldn't be surprised if our old foe reappears from time to time; it generally requires a prolonged effort to control this basic instinct.

When I decided to write and to give lectures, I was faced with the contradiction of wanting to communicate with others, while also being afraid of speaking in public. On many occasions I felt like saying, "Forget this, it's not worth the stress I'm causing myself." There was a battle raging within me, and I often thought that fear and worry were going to win. Frequently I would walk along the country road where I live, contemplating my dilemma. I have always had the desire to write—to communicate my thoughts through the written word. I know that writing and lecturing go hand in hand, and that speaking engagements are inevitable with the publication of a book. Finally, I decided to put absolute faith and confidence in my inner resources.

This has helped a great deal, enabling me to lecture without difficulty. There are still some occasions when I become anxious over public presentations, but I realize this is only the nervous anticipation that most people suffer from. In fact, I now consider such anticipation a healthy thing, if controlled, because it encourages one to be prepared and in good form during public engagements.

IV

THE medicine men and women in traditional cultures must have been keen observers of nature, able to interpret weather patterns and the behaviour of birds, animals, and other things important to their survival. After all, they spent their entire lives in close interaction with the natural landscape, were gifted with wisdom, and had a deep understanding of the cycles of nature. They were also master psychologists and the caretakers of ancient medicine knowledge. Because of this they were called upon to counsel, and their words were carefully regarded. In some instances the shaman would supervise the vision quests of young people who were about to become valuable adult members of society. These young people were seeking the guidance and help of spirit allies. The shaman would interpret the results of the quest as described to him, and give meaning to things otherwise difficult to understand. The vision quest was a means of facing fear—real or imagined—because it took great courage to go off alone, to fast, and to endure various hardships. In traditional cultures, the quest was a means of confronting fear, among other things. The shaman was there to advise, direct and help the participant to better understand the spirit world and the forces of nature, generally.

To face and to confront one's fear, or other obstacles in life, is to gain an increasing measure of freedom. The result is that external influences or internal habits have less ability to shape your life. You become increasingly open to change, to a willingness to move in directions that could change your circumstances for the better. Fear has lost its grip on your behaviour patterns and on the way you live your life. Nicholas Roerich remarked in his book *Shambhala*, that a person should "cast away ... that ridiculous fear which whispers, 'This is not for you.' One must be rid of that grey fear, mediocrity ... all is for you if you manifest the wish from a pure source" (p.151).

Exercise 2: *Exploring Your Past*

It is often valuable to examine the past. This is what you will do in this exercise. Go for a walk in a wooded area until you find a relaxing, pleasant environment where you can be alone with your thoughts. You should have a pen and notepad. When you find a pleasant location, sit, relax, and think about the things you have accomplished with your life. Make a list of your accomplishments, and try to determine those qualities of your character or personality that helped foster your success. On a second sheet of paper, list those things you feel you failed to achieve in the past. Be honest in your assessment, and include the things you actually made an effort to achieve, as well as those things that were in your dreams but were never quite attempted. Try to determine the factors in your environment and in yourself that prevented you from reaching those goals. Your examination will give you an understanding of the positive qualities of your personality, and an appreciation for those things you may want to change in the future.

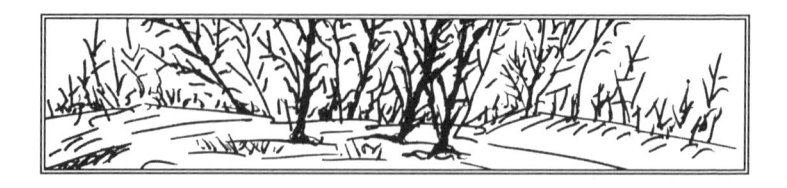

Chapter 2

THE DISCOVERY OF SPECIAL PLACES

THE cool breeze felt refreshing against my face as I ascended the narrow path through a thick cover of beech, maple, and other hardwoods. Everywhere nature's palette spread a blanket of autumn colour over the landscape. Occasionally, when there were breaks in the cover, I could see for miles over the canopy of forest covering much of this area of northern Maine. I had been hiking for only an hour, but already my legs were tired from the steep terrain of this mountainous country. But enthusiasm is stronger than fatigue! I wasn't about to be discouraged from my goal by anything short of a major confrontation with a bull moose. Katahdin was like an old dream waiting for fulfillment. I was there to experience the special mood of the mountains; to understand what was for me a foreign landscape.

Soon I broke the tree line, awestruck as my eyes scanned to the horizon mile after mile of autumn foliage. Mighty Katahdin stood directly in my path, like a guardian spirit protecting the soul of the land. My mind was infused with a wonderful feeling of well-being. Standing there, I understood why some people are haunted by that feeling, and why they often return to the mountains in search of it.

There is no doubt that mountains are special places of

immense benefit to those who approach them with respect, reverence, and a genuine love for the outdoor environment. I was reminded of Nicholas Roerich's words:

> *Where can one find such joy as when the sun is on the Himalayas; when the blue is more intense than sapphires; when from the far distance, the glaciers glitter as incomparable gems.* (Roerich, p. 41)

I have never witnessed first hand the spectacular, awe-inspiring majesty of the Himalayas—I can only imagine their beauty. But I can understand something of what Roerich felt, because I have stood on Kartahdin, looking west at peaks breaking the tree line all the way to the horizon. It is sometimes easy for us to forget that such wonderful places exist on earth; to be so caught up in everyday existence that we neglect those things that inspire and nourish the soul. We are blessed in that every area of the earth has places that affect the emotions and stimulate the imagination. Atlantic Canada is rich in such locations, due in part to its low population density, which affords people the luxury of enjoying nature in relative privacy. Indeed, privacy is very important, as I repeatedly stress. It allows us to play, dance, sing, cry, and do all the crazy things we would never do in public. In this way, privacy nourishes our mind, body, and spirit, allowing us to rest and recuperate from the everyday stress of modern society.

II

I HAVE considered the concept of "special places" for many years. My interest developed from a study of North American cultures and their recognition of sacred sites and energy centres. In many of those cultures, a place is sacred for several reasons: perhaps it is or was used for vision quests or religious rituals; it may be known for the spirit beings living there. One of my first opportunities to experience the power of a special energy centre came about during a visit to the American Southwest in 1987.

Just as the Himalayas symbolize the spiritual wisdom and inspiration that may be found in Asia, so too the American Southwest symbolizes the wisdom and inspiration that is part of the history and cultures of North America. Perhaps no place is more significant in this respect than Oak Creek Canyon, Arizona. Its high canyon walls of red sandstone are a virtual gallery on which the forces have sculptured designs of various shapes and sizes—reminders of the ancient figures of Hopi and Anasazi spirit beings. Similarly wonderful is the way the changing light of that place affects those images as the sun moves across the sky towards sunset.

Many people consider Oak Creek Canyon a centre of high energy concentration or, in New Age parlance, an "energy vortex centre." Those people are of diverse philosophical orientation, and include students of so-called New Age teachings, or those involved in metaphysical studies, as well as students of Native American cultures. The depth of the belief in Oak Creek Canyon as an energy centre became evident to me upon my arrival in Arizona. At the time I was a volunteer worker at the Hopi Traditionals' Center in Flagstaff. Special areas such as Oak Creek Canyon were sometimes the subject of discussion among the volunteers and, occasionally, among the Hopi. My curiosity was aroused to the point where I was determined to experience the area on foot.

III

The drive from Flagstaff to Oak Creek is impressive, especially the forests of ponderosa pine, which are evident everywhere. Approaching Oak Creek, the road winds snakelike down the canyon walls, continuously twisting and turning back on itself. We arrived in the canyon on a hot July afternoon. While my friends had come to swim in the creek, I was there to climb Cathedral Rock, a large rock formation immediately above the creek. The crest of the formation has large wind-sculptured pillows of red sandstone that stand like silent guardians.

The temperature was 30° Celsius when I began my climb. With each step, dust rose from the parched soil beneath my feet. Occasionally, small lizards dashed over the ground, seemingly delighted that they were not far removed from the cool water of the creek. Such numbers of lizards were foreign to me, as was the dry soil of the landscape. This definitely isn't Atlantic Canada, I thought, as I moved carefully, always on the alert for rattlesnakes. In fact, I was probably more careful than I needed to be. I figured this was justified since I knew little about the behaviour of rattlers or other snakes of the Southwest. As well, my friends in Flagstaff had advised me not to step blindly over fallen trees or other objects and, when climbing, never to place my hand on a ledge or flat surface before checking that there were no rattlers sunbathing there.

The climb from the base of Cathedral Rock to the shelf jutting out from a vertical rock face towering above me was difficult. The soil was loose and unreliable under my feet. Fortunately I was able to climb without the aid of ropes, pegs, or other equipment. The shelf itself was several metres

13

wide and very sandy, with the occasional small plant or shrub growing there. I stopped to examine a shrub, about a metre high, with thorns on its bark. The plant was totally unlike anything I could remember seeing before. I regretted not having brought along a plant reference book. Following the shelf, I came to a shallow cave carved into the vertical rock face. It was about two metres high, somewhat wider than that, and extended back into the rock about three metres. Crawling into the cave, I found it gave excellent shelter from the heat of the sun, although I remember shuddering at the thought of having such a massive amount of rock over my head.

The shelf, I discovered, made its way around Cathedral Rock to a break in the vertical wall, which allowed me to approach the sculptured guardians. Leaving the cave, I was alerted to the sound of birds and astonished to see seven eagles circling directly overhead. It was an emotional and humbling experience, although not as humbling as when I found myself in the centre of that special place, standing on a table rock between those towering guardians. The table rock was very flat, as if it had been sculptured and placed there with purpose. The view was breathtaking. As I looked out over Oak Creek Canyon, I realized that these were special moments, and that I would continue to gain strength from them for the remainder of my life.

Retracing my steps towards Oak Creek, I was startled by a sudden vertical drop in the landscape. Visually it seemed to me that the landscape had changed, but, logically, I reasoned that somehow I must have taken the wrong path. The drop was at least fifteen metres and impossible to descend without ropes or the knowledge of an experienced rock climber. I had no choice but to backtrack and find another route down to

Oak Creek. While considering the situation, I noticed a "wash" that seemed to run all the way down to the vicinity of the creek. Stepping carefully over rocks, some of which must have measured a metre in diameter, I ascended the wash. I imagine that most of those rocks were deposited during flash floods. I visualized a flood rushing down the wash, carrying away everything in its path, including rocks, soil, insects, snakes, lizards, and other small animals. Snakes were uppermost on my mind—I figured the wash was a good place to find them. It was certainly the last place I wanted to be, but the quickest way to descend Cathedral Rock.

As fate would have it, I soon located the shelf that I had followed on my ascent. It was about thirty metres to my right. Moving quickly, I soon intercepted my old footprints in the dry soil, and made a swift retreat to the creek, periodically answering shouts from my friends, who were becoming concerned for my safety.

I remember thinking at the time that, despite the beauty of the place and its spiritual nourishment, I hadn't felt any particular effects on my physical body, as I might have expected from such a special energy centre. On the other hand, I realized that those vibrations, if they are magnetic, are quite subtle, and no more noticeable than the force of gravity, for example, which, while profound in its effects, is simply taken for granted by most of us. However, I did notice definite effects the following day, and for a week afterwards. I felt fantastic. It was like I was running on a highly charged battery. I am convinced that there is something very special about the Cathedral Rock area.

IV

I BELIEVE there are special energy centres in eastern North America, including the Atlantic provinces. The concept of special energy centres may be difficult to accept, since it challenges the way we normally view the landscape, but is it really so impossible to imagine? Consider Cape Blomidon, in Nova Scotia. Here is an area sacred to the Mi'kmaq people, steeped in tradition and legend, especially legends pertaining to Glooscap, the great cultural hero of the Mi'kmaq. If you visit Cape Blomidon, you will certainly be impressed with its beauty and splendour. However, if you have some background knowledge of its legendary past—and respect for Native traditions associated with the place—you will most certainly come away feeling you have touched and walked upon sacred earth. It will leave you with lasting impressions, similar to those you might have if you visited a beautiful cathedral or walked upon the holy sites in the Middle East.

Related to the subject of special energy centres is the question of what effects minerals have on human beings. We are well aware of the devastating effects of uranium radiation, but what are the effects of minerals such as iron, silver, and gold? What rates of vibrations do they release and what is their influence on humans and other life forms? Also, does gender influence those vibrations? Do men and women relate differently to the earth's influences? Such questions may seem vague and difficult to explore, but they are worth considering.

I am especially interested in the influence gold has on the human emotions. I believe it affects people in different ways, depending on personality types. In fact, it is possible that gold and other precious minerals are present at special energy centres. This is strictly a personal hypothesis, based largely on the fact that one of my special places lies in a gold-bearing area. It is a place that exerts a strong influence on me, both mentally and emotionally.

This raises the question of how to locate high-energy centres in our own area of the world. There are several ways to approach this question. While hiking, always be on the alert for possible high-energy locations. Explore an area thoroughly and, when you happen upon a location you feel has special features, remain there for a period of time. Revisit the place frequently, and note whether you feel especially invigorated. If you sense positive effects, try to verify your first impressions. Have other people visit the same area and record their feelings. Tell several friends that you have found a special place and want to take them there. Or, keep your friends in the dark about your discovery, but take them to the location and note whether they are especially enthused about the area, either during the visit or afterwards. It is beneficial to network with people who have a similar interest in special places. In this way you will be able to share information on several of your favourite locations, including energy centres. Finally, create and use affirmations pertaining to special places. Affirm that you will discover places of special value. Continue to affirm this on a daily basis until you dream of such locations, or are intuitively guided to them.

Special energy centres, such as Cathedral Rock, are difficult to locate, but the effort of searching for them is rewarding and therapeutic in itself. Of course, it is much easier to access places that, although not energy centres, are conducive to meditation and affect the emotions in a positive manner. Often it is as simple as noting those places that attract you, or for which you have a great affinity. For instance, I have a special attraction for the Leipsigaek gold fields (also known as Maliepsigaek), an area west of Bridgewater, Nova Scotia, which I have visited frequently over the past 30 years. The place inspires me, and I have learned to use it for therapeutic purposes. I love to hike in that area, to absorb everything I possibly can from the landscape, and to visit the many places there that soothe the emotions or inspire the creative urges within me.

If we wish to reconnect to mother earth, and to maximize the benefits of outdoor therapy, it is important to discover such places for ourselves. These locations become our own personal places where we can seek privacy and healing in our lives. In the following pages there are a variety of exercises to use in conjunction with these locations. Remember, it is important to locate your own special places. Such places may consist of several square miles where you feel especially comfortable, joyful, and inspired. Or, they could be small, specific locations. Begin by discovering the small, specific locations, which are often found within the larger special areas. Visit them on a regular basis. During your visits, consider how they affect your emotions, or whether they stimulate your creative urges. Do they help to relieve the stress in your life? Or, is there an area that seems especially to promote relaxation and peace of mind? After careful consideration and experimentation, select one or two of these locations as your special places, where you will go to meditate and practise the exercises in complete privacy.

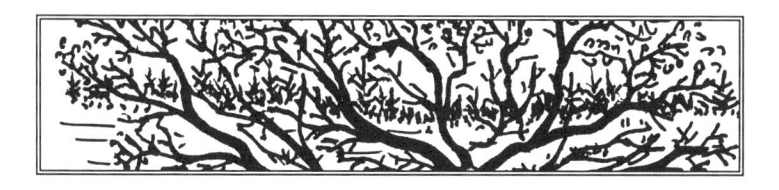

Chapter 3

USING OUR SPECIAL PLACES

SPECIAL places are central to my relationship with the landscape. There are a number of areas in my immediate environment that I frequent often, not only because I enjoy hiking there, but because these places are especially healing to mind and body. These are places where we may engage the landscape in dialogue; by this I mean that we may get to know an area especially well, how its mood changes with the weather, the time of day, or with the seasons. We may become acquainted with the animals and birds that frequent the area—their behaviour patterns, trails, and flight paths—as well as with the nature of the insect life. Then the place begins to assume the aura of an old friend whom we know especially well. Special places are like old friends whom we can visit with our problems, and in whom we find both support and solutions. It is this kind of intimacy which we should seek with our special places.

Some systems of self-development apply the same principle of special places on a strictly imaginative basis; they recommend the visualization of a "special room" or place in which to perform various exercises. One can then "return" to this room to practise exercises. Undoubtedly this approach is effective, especially if practised over a period of time, as we soon learn to associate the visualized room with a particular state of mind.

However, I believe that using places in the physical environment for visualization practice is more effective than using places created in the mind. This is because in addition to the mental benefits you receive from repeated use of a familiar location for your exercises, the physical landscape is naturally pleasing and special. Let's face it, simply walking or relaxing in a pleasant outdoor environment has wonderful therapeutic benefits, without the necessity of mental exertion in any form.

I am especially attracted to isolated rock-strewn landscapes. Rocks are magical in their ability to create particular moods through a combination of shape, colour, texture, and pattern. If the soil is right, there is usually plant cover such as teaberry and crowberry. Often the rocks, especially if they are granites, will be partially covered with mosses and lichens. For me, those places are especially conducive to deep reflection and inspiration. In this landscape, I allow my imagination to run wild, to envisage how it must have looked a hundred, a thousand, or a hundred thousand years ago. Here, it is easy to imagine that nature spirits are hiding in the crevices of rocks or behind certain boulders, or that fairies dance their circles on the soft blankets of moss.

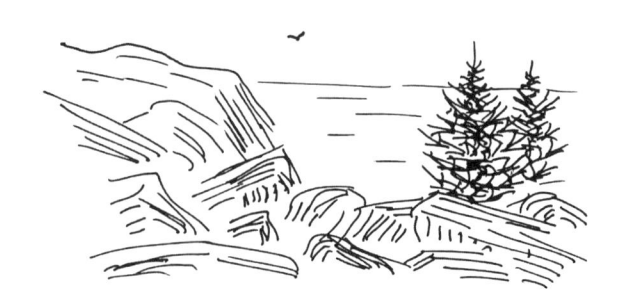

Exercise 3: The Life History of Objects

Find a landscape with interesting rock formations. This should be easy if you live near the ocean, since shorelines are good places to find unusual rock formations. Lakes are also good places in this respect. Walk the area and determine what emotions it conveys to you. After you have thoroughly familiarized yourself with the location, choose a place to sit. Place your palms on the rock face on which you are sitting. Relax your mind and focus on your hands. Imagine that you are going to read the life history of the rock. Visualize the vibrations coming from it through your hands, up your arms, and into your head. When you have attained a strong visualization, let your mind go blank. Watch the screen of your mind, and note whatever impressions begin to appear. Do not hold onto them, but let them come and go freely. After five to ten minutes, open your eyes and consider whether you feel the impressions shed light on the history of the rock.

II

One morning four ravens sat at the edge of the desert waiting for the sun to rise. They had been there all night and the dew was like beads of quicksilver on their wings. Their eyes were closed and they were as still as the cracks in the desert floor ... At first light their bodies swelled and their eyes flashed purple. When the dew dried on their wings they lifted off from the desert floor.

Barry Holstun Lopez
Desert Notes, Reflections in the Eye of a Raven, p. 5

I AM convinced that the characteristic that people refer to as "patience" is everywhere present in nature. It is present in the spider as it waits to trap a fly or an insect in its web. It is present in the crow or a raven as it sits on a tree branch scanning the horizon for its mate. This quality of nature is implied in the life of a rock as it weathers and erodes over thousands of years. It is also implied in the growth of a forest, or a single blade of grass. There are many other such examples in nature, evident to the discerning eye.

How many of us have considered the value of patience in our own lives? Or, if we recognize its value, how many of us have consciously taken the time to cultivate patience? Few of us realize that the natural world offers valuable instruction on patience. I learned this during my teenage years from a spider. I was sitting in the basement of my home, trying to cool off on a hot July afternoon, when I noticed a large, brown spider near the entrance steps. It had woven its web between two rocks. Its size caught my attention, and I wondered if it were poisonous, and wished I had a field manual on spiders.

There were numerous other webs on the basement wall, reminding me that perhaps spiders were community-minded insects rather than the solitary creatures I had always imagined them to be. I thought how interesting it would be to study spider behaviour, and realized how little I actually knew about them. I even mused about going to university and specializing in the study of insects. When my attention returned to the spider, it was still sitting motionless on its web. I was curious about what it would do next. I must have observed the creature for 30 minutes before I realized that it wasn't going anywhere, and would probably stay right where it was for the rest of the day.

The spider gave me a lesson in patience that afternoon. It was waiting for the slightest vibration of its web, telling it that something, perhaps a fly, was trapped there. For the next several months, I would occasionally go down to the basement to visit that spider. Whenever I found it sitting Buddha-like on its web, I would attempt to emulate its practice, even trying to sit still until the spider moved. Well, I never achieved my goal, but my patience did improve significantly because of my relationship with the spider—a teacher of patience and stillness.

Exercise 4: Patience

This exercise explores the value of "patience" in our lives, and requires 15 to 20 minutes. Consider your life during the past month, and write down those occasions when greater patience would have benefited you. When you are finished, examine the list and determine whether your situation would be different today had you exercised more patience in your affairs. For example, would results have been significantly different in a business deal or a relationship?

Exercise 5: Observing Clouds

On a cloudy day, go to your special place and assume a comfortable position. If you wish, take a cushion or something that will assure your comfort and relaxation. Relax. Determine this day to befriend the clouds and make them your allies. You can use the clouds to develop patience.

Observe the clouds as they float across the sky. Imagine each cloud as a problem or an event in your life. Notice how the clouds are temporary objects in our line of vision, and how they float away from us. Realize that problems and events in life are as temporary and fleeting as the clouds passing across your field of vision. Know that if you approach the events in your life in a relaxed and patient manner, they will lose much of their power to affect or disturb you. You will feel less panic and fear, and realize the fleeting nature of events.

Remain relaxed and observe each cloud as it crosses your field of vision. Note the shape, colours, size, and other characteristics of the clouds. This quiet observation will develop your patience if you persist in its practice. (Suggested time: 30 minutes.)

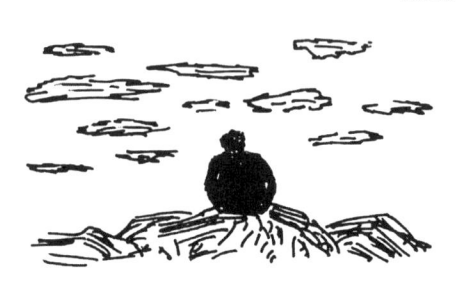

Exercise 6: Patience and Observation

Visit your special place and assume a comfortable position. As in the previous exercise, you may wish to use a cushion or a chair. This exercise will stretch the limits of your patience. It is effective in improving your ability to sit still, to observe, and to become more aware of the environment around you.

Relax. Examine the environment, noting the different shapes, colours, animals, birds, insects, kinds of plant life, and types of rocks. Note the many new things you are able to observe about your special place that you failed to see before. Continue this process. When you feel you have carefully scanned the environment, close your eyes and search for sounds that you may have missed.

This will test your ability to observe and sit relaxed for a period of time. Slowly take a deep breath, exhale, then repeat. Continue to observe your surroundings. Pretend you are a bird; perhaps an eagle, hawk, owl, raven, or crow. Watch for movement, signs of life, or any indication of things you may have missed previously. Do this until you are satisfied that you have exhausted everything in the environment on this particular day. (Suggested time: 30 to 40 minutes.)

III

*In concentration, the consciousness is
held to a single image; the whole attention
of the knower is fixed on a single point,
without wavering or swerving.*
Annie Besant
Thought Power: Its Control and Practice, p. 79

CONCENTRATION is closely allied with patience. A person who sits in front of an easel and executes a meticulous painting of a flower or a finely detailed portrait must not only have skill as a painter, but also have full concentration on the task at hand. He or she must also have a good deal of patience to correct mistakes along the way, or to avoid shortcuts that would make the painting less accomplished. In today's Western society, many people are short of both patience and concentration. Fortunately, these are qualities that can be cultivated and improved, regardless of our age. The ability to concentrate allows us to enjoy our hobbies, to set goals with a greater likelihood of accomplishment, and even to realize greater benefits from friendships. For instance, many of us have had conversations with people who don't seem to take the time to listen to what we are saying. Their minds are elsewhere and they interrupt our sentences. They lack basic listening skills. Both patience and concentration are essential to the art of listening to others.

A number of methods are available to enhance one's ability to concentrate on a given subject or object. Those methods, many of which are excellent, are readily available in the form of books, cassettes, and videos. In this book, we focus on nature, using the natural landscape and our physical surroundings to develop the power of concentration.

Of course it doesn't matter how many books we read, videos we view, or lectures we attend, if we don't practise persistence. This is an important consideration. We need a relaxed persistence. Performing an exercise once will not achieve much. You must persist, but never in a tense or strained manner. Do not hurry. Always try to maintain a relaxed approach to the exercises given in this book.

There have been many instances in my life where I've lacked the persistence to continue with a practice or the pursuit of a goal. For instance, I very much admire the life and teachings of Paramahansa Yogananda. He was one of the first Masters of Yoga to bring the ancient teachings to the Western world, including North America. Yet, in the past, I've lacked the discipline to practise Yoga exercises and meditation on a regular basis. Still, I have persisted, and now I am more able to apply myself to these practices.

The series of exercises that follow are given to improve concentration. Each of the exercises should be tried at least twice. Later, choose a couple of exercises to practise on a regular basis.

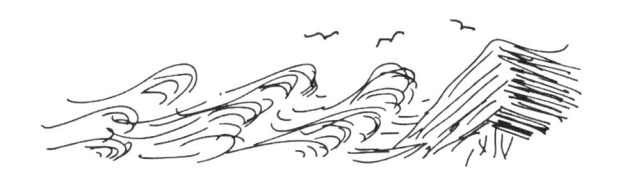

Exercise 7: Observing the Waves

Visit the ocean or a lake to find a private place where you will not be disturbed. Sit in a comfortable position, relax, and slowly take several deep breaths. Close your eyes. Concentrate on the natural inflow and outflow of your breath. Do this for approximately five minutes; then, opening your eyes, notice the peaceful, relaxed feeling.

Focus your attention on the waves; then, on a single wave, watching it move towards the shore. Follow the wave until it splashes on the rocks or dissipates along the shoreline. Maintain a relaxed attitude as you calmly observe the wave. Examine its characteristics—continue to do this with individual wave movements. If you become restless, reaffirm your calm approach and continue with the exercise. (Suggested time: 20 to 30 minutes.)

Exercise 8: The Crow as Ally

In this exercise, the crow will be your ally and assist you in developing your concentration. You must walk until you find a crow perched on a tree or on some other object. As you walk, try to concentrate on discovering just the right crow for your purpose. However, be sure to remain at a safe distance, so you won't disturb the crow. There will be occasions when you do not locate a crow to observe. However, you must give yourself at least 30 minutes to an hour to do so. It is important to concentrate on finding a crow. This in itself will strengthen your ability to concentrate, so that even if you fail to locate a crow, the exercise will be beneficial.

Once you have located a crow, assume a comfortable position and relax, slowly taking several deep breaths. Focus your attention on the crow. Do not think of anything else, and try not to allow your attention to be diverted to other objects or creatures in the environment. Calmly focus on the crow. If you are fortunate, your observations will give you insight into the process of concentration—you will discover where you are weak, and realize what you must do to improve your ability to concentrate. Also, you will gain a greater appreciation for crows, and realize that it is possible to learn many things from them. In fact, as you observe the crow, ask yourself what it can teach you about patience and concentration. (Suggested time: 30 minutes.)

Exercise *9*: *Concentration on an Object*

Visit your special place, assume a comfortable position, and relax. Look about the environment and find an object that interests you. The object can be a rock, a tree, or something else. Calmly observe the object. Allow yourself to become absorbed in the study of the object, even to the point where you forget about the other elements in your environment, or about yourself. (Suggested time: 20 to 30 minutes.)

Exercise **10**: *Focus on Sounds*

Take a walk or a drive into the country, and find a place where there is a variety of natural sounds. Those sounds can be the buzzing of bees, birds singing, running water, waves splashing on rocks, frogs peeping, or a breeze blowing through the trees. Find a comfortable, private place to sit. Relax and take several deep breaths. Close your eyes and listen to the sounds. Choose a particular sound and focus your attention on that sound to the exclusion of other sounds. After several minutes, shift your attention to a second sound, and proceed until you have listened to each of the sounds in turn. Finally, choose a favourite sound, and concentrate your attention on that sound for ten minutes. (Suggested time: 30 to 40 minutes.)

Exercise **11**: *Tactile Impressions*

In this exercise you are to focus all your concentration on tactile impressions—on the sense of touch. Visit your special place and examine the plant life there. Choose a plant or small tree that interests you. Assume a position next to the plant, breathe deeply and hold the breath for a few seconds. Exhale. Repeat twice more. Relax and examine the plant visually. Then, close your eyes and gently examine the plant with your fingers. Concentrate on your sense of touch—the impressions coming to you through your fingers. Feel the texture of the plant, the shape of its leaves, the thickness and texture of the stem and side branches. Hold the plant. Notice other impressions that register in your mind. (Suggested time: 20 to 30 minutes.)

Exercise 12: Your Special Place on the Full Moon

The main purpose of this exercise is to train yourself to concentrate with singlemindedness. Proceed to your special place on the night of a full moon. Find a comfortable place to sit. Relax. Examine the environment in the moonlight. After several minutes, focus your sight on a distant point—hold the sight on that point, but do not strain your eyes. Focus in a relaxed manner and blink your eyes whenever necessary. As you sit, pay attention to visual impressions that might arise. After the exercise, relax, look about you, and examine the impressions and feelings of your special place under moonlight conditions. Notice how the mood differs from the daylight hours. (Suggested maximum time for concentrated focus: 15 minutes.)

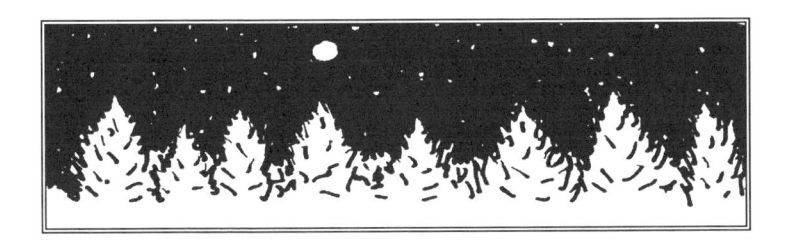

Chapter 4

COPING WITH STRESS THE NATURAL WAY

STRESSFUL situations are a daily occurrence in today's fast-paced world. This is a major problem in modern Western society—certainly a primary factor in a large number of mental and physical health problems, which in turn sends health care and insurance-related costs skyrocketing. Stress can be rooted in the pressure to perform on certain occasions, or the pressure to maintain certain standards on a continuous basis. For instance, consider the enormous stress that air traffic controllers or pilots experience. Similarly, school teachers are under an increasing amount of stress as they strive to educate children in a highly competitive world; add to this the many disciplinary problems confronting teachers and you have a recipe for both stress and nervous breakdown. Again, consider the problems parents face—in particular, single parents—as they struggle to raise their children while functioning within the pressures of various kinds of relationships. Two-parent families face many of the same problems, with marital partnerships often stressed to the brink of collapse.

But the point I want to emphasize is that we are not helpless in the face of stressful circumstances. There are things we can do for ourselves to better cope with life's pressures. I am not advocating self-treatment for serious mental or emotional problems, although, even here, informed self therapy in conjunction with professional help can be very beneficial. Self-treatment can be empowering and give one a sense of control over one's own wellness. This alone may contribute significantly to self-esteem and psychological health.

Some may question whether a naturalist, such as myself, should discuss the problem of stress, when such subjects are clearly in the domain of health professionals. My answer is simply that I believe persons outside the mainstream of the health professions have important things to say concerning human health and welfare. As we move through our lives, gaining experience in earth's schoolhouse, we acquire valuable insights that should be shared with others. As a naturalist, I think I have gained an understanding of the natural landscape that I have an obligation to share; part of this understanding relates to our well-being as living, conscious beings functioning within the environment.

There is a close relationship between how we feel, our moods, and our living environment. There are things we can do to make any environment or living atmosphere a happier and more joyous experience. I know an artist who applied this philosophy to his life at a time when he lacked the initiative to paint. He felt indifferent to painting, lacked inspiration, and was unable to find satisfying subject matter. This landscape painter specialized in panoramic scenes of valleys, fields, and fast-flowing rivers. He has a house in the country on about 20 acres of land. One day he decided that, rather than trying to paint while he was in such a rut, he would apply his studio time differently. He began to take morning walks instead of painting. However, his walks were different. He imagined and conceived his home as the hub on a spoked wheel, and each morning he began his walk in a different direction. Occasionally the direction would be such that he would follow roads, while at other times he would leave his home and go directly into the forest, walking slowly and paying careful attention to the sights and sounds around him. It wasn't long before he brought along a sketchbook, and made brief representations of things that interested him, always noting colours, shadows, and the direction of the light.

This simple activity aroused his desire to paint again, even changing somewhat his usual subject matter. While he still continued to paint the panoramic scenery, much of his work began to focus on small things within the landscape, such as moss-covered stumps, rock formations, and birds. His story is a good example of how we can take the initiative to overcome problems—such as lack of inspiration or artistic blocks—to perform again at a high level of creativity.

The point we should remember is that our creativity can manifest itself in many forms. For instance, we are verbal creatures, able to use the "spoken word" to change our experience of the world around us. This verbal gift enables us to interact with each other in complex ways to bring about positive changes in our neighbourhoods and relationships. Another important consideration is that none of us views the world as it actually exists. Our vision of the world is coloured and filtered through our minds. Each of us has our own unique conscious realization of the vibrations from the world around us—the vibrations of physical existence. It is up to us to shape this realization in constructive ways, to the best of our ability. I am speaking in particular of the small things we can do to make our lives more fulfilling. For instance, taking

30 minutes daily for a brisk walk; reading a good book over lunch hour, or meditating for ten minutes each day are some of the ways we can improve our lives. Small changes can result in a very positive reorientation in our daily schedule of activities, and can be a precursor to healthy adjustments in lifestyle.

Individuals who find themselves in oppressive relationships may discover through analysis that their self-expression is smothered, and that most of their activities are geared towards the domineering partner. This is a good example of a situation where small changes in personal activities are appropriate. In this way, one is able to gradually change the nature of a relationship to a point where a healthy balance is possible. Of course, a partner may be so inflexible that they totally oppose such restructuring activities. In this case, a reasonable course of action is to seek professional counselling.

II

OUR bodies and minds are exposed to many poisons on a daily basis. For example, affluents released into the atmosphere may cause an assortment of problems from general environmental sensitivities to lung disorders or tumours, among other things. We are also regularly exposed to dangerous viruses. Similarly, whenever a person walks into the forest they are exposed to a vast continuum of life, including plants and mushrooms, many of which are poisonous, even fatal to ingest. Finally, there are the truly invisible poisons, things that cannot be examined under a microscope. They are the mental poisons, including fear, negative thought patterns, and stress. These poisons do not always occur separately; stress can be rooted in deep-seated fear or simply in the fear of performing a certain activity. If we develop the ability to cope with fear, we are able to rid ourselves of much daily stress.

Considerable stress is also faced daily by physically and mentally challenged individuals. These persons are routinely the victims of discrimination or of misunderstanding, of being considered "different" from other people, and of having to meet challenges in everyday life that many people take for granted. As a youngster growing up in the 1950s, I used to resent those occasions when someone called me "the crippled boy." I hated it. It was like a virus attacking my mental health. In those days, people were not sensitive to such mental pain. If you were a person with a physical handicap, you were "the crippled person." It was even worse for people with permanent brain damage or serious mental problems. Those persons were identified as "morons" or "lunatics," fit only for an asylum. This was the prevailing attitude.

We must take it upon ourselves to combat both fear and stress; to promote personal growth, happiness, and joy. These things cannot be provided in our lives by tranquilizers, sedatives, or antidepressant drugs. Such drugs are temporary stop-gap measures, except where they are absolutely necessary. I do not mean to imply that persons with serious illnesses should give up drug therapy. Obviously there are many people who must take drugs for physical or mental problems. However, there are also large numbers of people who are quick to take tranquilizers, sedatives, antidepressants and the like for minor problems, without exploring alternative ways of dealing with their difficulties. Ultimately, personal growth, freedom, and health are gained by living a balanced life without the aid of drugs, and by knowing how to use other non-addictive tools to maintain that balance. Those tools (for instance, the exercises in this book) will encourage us to go forward to experience those things that make life truly beautiful. If we affirm to do this, nature will be our ally.

Aside from specific exercises, there are a number of steps we can take to handle stress and stress-related problems. Some of these are so simple, one would hardly think they need mentioning. However, as is often the case, the simple steps are overlooked. Occasionally they should be reaffirmed or given greater emphasis in our daily lives. Some of those steps are given below.

1. *It is very beneficial to practise meditation* if you are a person who is prone to stress, or have to face stressful situations on a daily basis. Find a form of meditation that is attractive to you and compatible with your lifestyle. Practise it regularly.

2. *If you are a highly stressed individual, it is important to slow down,* to realize that the fast-paced pattern of your life is contributing to your problems. Slow down or take time out from your schedule to consider the dangers that stress poses to your health, and the worry that you may be causing your family. Consider to what extent external environmental circumstances are controlling your life. Ask yourself these questions: To what extent am I making the decisions in my life? Are outside influences such as job, friends, and social pressures constantly driving my decisions?

You must make time for yourself, your friends, and for your family.

Simplicity, simplicity, simplicity! I say, let your affairs be as two or three, and not a hundred or a thousand; instead of a million count half a dozen, and keep your account on a thumbsnail.
                    Henry David Thoreau, *Walden* in Krutch (ed.)
                    Thoreau: Walden and Other Writings, p. 173.

3. *Take the time* to consider what you enjoy most about nature and the outdoors; apply it to its fullest!

4. *Concentrate on those things you like to do,* especially those hobbies or pursuits that tend to make you relax, or physical activities that release tension. Also, if you analyse yourself, you may discover all kinds of little things you have done in the past to cope with stress. You can apply this knowledge and experience on a regular basis.

5. *Begin to reach out and cultivate a good relationship with another person.* This will bring you happiness, enabling you to better cope with difficulties in life. It is wonderful to have someone special in your life with whom you can confide whatever you wish. Also, socialize more often; join others for tea, coffee, shopping, or hiking.

6. *Take regular walks.* Walking is beneficial to physical and mental health, and for the removal of tension from the body. If you are unable to walk and move about freely, perhaps you can use a wheelchair for regular outings. Whatever your situation, attempt to exercise or involve your body in a manner compatible with your physical health and life circumstances.

7. *Cultivate a love of reading, writing, sketching, or painting.* These are things you can do at home, or almost any place that strikes your fancy.

Exercise 13: *In the Protection of Your Special Place*

Consider your special place a refuge or sanctuary where you go to relax and unwind from stressful situations. You must treat your special place as an ally, a friend; a place safe from stress, worry, and the storms of life. There are many ways to reinforce this concept of "special place" or sanctuary, but none of the methods are more effective than ritual and ceremony. Try performing the following ritual involving the scattering of tobacco during visits to your special place. Tobacco has an important ceremonial function in many traditional cultures. Aside from the plants in the genus *Nicotiana*, other plants or combinations of plants are also used. For example, the *kinnickanick* used by North American Native peoples is a combination of several plants; the plants vary somewhat among the different Nations.

In my opinion, commercial tobacco should not be used for ceremonial or spiritual purposes, since it is not planted, grown, harvested, or prepared in a prayerful manner. One alternative is to grow your own tobacco; another is to collect and dry wild plants and tree barks, and combine them in a tobacco-like mixture. Again, if a particular plant is special to you, you may want to use it for sacred purposes.

This ritual should be performed in the following way: facing east, scatter a small portion of tobacco, thinking as you do so that you are sealing the east from detrimental influences, and inviting joyful, loving energy. Follow with the south, west, and north directions in consecutive order. When you have completed the tobacco scattering ritual, feel satisfied and confident that you are in a protected, healing sanctuary, and that you may proceed with any exercise or action necessary for the healing of your body and mind. Use this ceremony on a regular basis. Eventually you will find that it promotes a positive psychological mood for whatever you plan to do within your special place.

Exercise 14: Wind Cleansing
(This exercise should be practised in windy or breezy conditions, or when there is a steady breeze.)

> *Attention is the key.... It is not a simple*
> *physical change but rather the state of*
> *mind that is the key to health.... This state*
> *has been called ... "restful alertness"....*
> *Like the ice breaking free in a spring thaw*
> *... stresses seem to melt.... Paying attention to*
> *Stress in a relaxed state transforms it.*
>
> Marilyn Ferguson,
> The Aquarian Conspiracy, pp. 250-51

Visit your special place. Choose a location where you can comfortably stand, sit, or recline, and where the wind strikes your body. Sit, relax, close your eyes, and concentrate on the sound of the wind as it blows over your special place. Feel it against your face—raise your hands, palms into the wind, and feel its impressions. (Suggested time: five minutes.)

Assume a standing position (eyes open or closed), facing into the wind. If it is a warm day, remove unnecessary clothing (as much clothing as modesty will allow). Slowly inhale through your nostrils, concentrating on the air as it fills the lungs. Do not inhale to the point where it becomes uncomfortable. If you have a health problem, such as a weak heart, or any other problem that deep breathing may aggravate, do not attempt this part of the exercise. The exercise will give beneficial results without deep breathing. Hold for five seconds, visualizing the blood becoming invigorated and highly charged by the fresh influx of oxygen and life force. Repeat three times. Resume regular breathing and remain standing. Feel the fresh air against your body. Slowly rotate your body clockwise, allowing the wind to touch each part as you turn. Imagine the wind purifying your body and mind.

Recline with your feet into the wind (a reclining lawn chair is good for this purpose). Close your eyes. Allow every muscle in your body to relax, beginning with your toes. Relax each part of your body in turn. Try to become like a dry leaf in the wind, eliminating all bodily tension and casting aside your cares and worries. Imagine the wind cleansing your body and mind of all its stress poisons. Remain in this position for five to ten minutes. Finally, open your eyes and slowly move each part of your body, beginning with your toes and ending with your head.

Exercise *15*: *Transference—Shamanic Removal of Toxins*

Begin the day with the idea that you are going to rid your mind and body of all stress-related toxins. After breakfast you should hike, walk, or drive to a lake; it can be a familiar lake or one you have never frequented prior to this occasion. The purpose of visiting this place is to find a rock into which you can transfer your stress, worry, and fear. You must walk the shore of the lake until you find a rock that you feel will be suitable for this purpose. Allow your intuition and good judgement to be your guide. When you find a suitable rock, wash it in the water and let it dry.

Transfer your stress and related problems to the rock in two stages: first, take the rock and move it slowly over every part of your body. It does not have to touch the body; the important thing is to visualize the rock gathering the stress and other toxins as you move it over your body. Second, hold the rock in your hands, concentrating on it to the exclusion of everything else. Focus completely on the rock. After about one minute of concentration, visualize any remaining toxins from your body and mind going into the rock. When you are satisfied that all the toxins are removed, take the rock and toss it as far as you can out into the water. At the same time, shout "They are gone!" As the rock disappears into the lake, imagine the water purifying the rock and destroying all the toxins. (Repeat this exercise often to aid in stress-related or other personal problems.)

Exercise 16: The White Cloud

Lie down, close your eyes, and relax. Try to imagine a fluffy white cloud forming under your body. The cloud is larger than your body. As it forms, imagine it lifting you from the ground. Visualize yourself becoming very light as the cloud rises into the air carrying you with it. Try to feel the motion as you float through the air. Enjoy the ride and release all your cares. Later, when you are ready, feel the cloud slowly sinking to the earth again. When you are safely on the ground, the cloud dissolves. Get up, stretch, and go about your business. You may want to do this exercise often, for the peaceful state it provides.

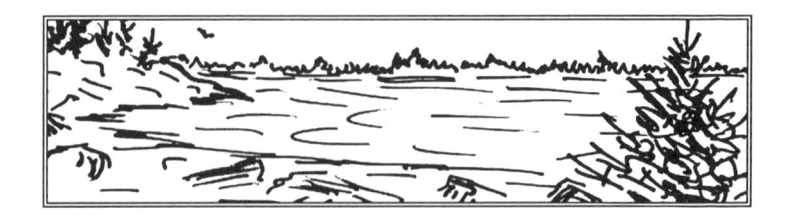

Chapter 5

EXPANDING OUR HORIZONS

SEVERAL years ago I chose the rugged landscape around Leipsigaek Lake to search for a "talking stick." I was convinced that I would find one there. The area has an abundance of bayberry, huckleberry, and lambkill bushes, interspersed with carpets of crowberry weaving itself over and around the myriad of odd-shaped boulders scattered throughout. Of all those plants, it was the huckleberry that challenged me that day. Ordinarily, I love huckleberries. Yet on this day it seemed they were especially difficult to manoeuvre through. Only grudgingly did they give way to the forward motion of my legs. Often I was forced to high-step through them or to take circuitous routes around the masses of bushes. Even so, I remember tripping once and landing face-down in the bushes. Adding to my difficulty was the heat of a July afternoon and the swarm of deerflies circling my head.

I searched everywhere for the talking stick, without finding anything that even remotely resembled what I had envisaged. I was disappointed, confused, hot, thirsty, and having a miserable time. Finally, after walking for what seemed like hours, I decided to relax in the shade of a grove of poplar trees. Lying there, I suddenly realized that perhaps I shouldn't be looking for the talking stick. Perhaps I wasn't approaching the problem correctly. I realized it was okay to be intent on finding the stick, and that the "intent" was enough. I was simply trying too hard and making a number of rational judgements on what constituted a good talking stick. Rather, I determined simply to allow myself to be guided to a stick. Interestingly enough, having made a decision on how to proceed, the remainder of my day was much more enjoyable, with the huckleberry seeming less antagonistic. Incidentally, I left that place without my talking stick.

In Native cultures, the talking stick used within the circle is a symbol for people gathered together, sharing feelings, emotions, ideas, and beliefs with each other in a supportive environment. It is an egalitarian circle of people, where each person has an opportunity to hold the stick, expressing thoughts on any given matter. In this way, people reach a consensus on a subject. This equality of the people and sharing of purpose is the power of the talking stick, which, in turn, supports the sacred nature and solidarity of the circle. The circle is implicit in nature and is expressive of nature's sacred laws.

II

I BELIEVE it is important to have personal dreams and goals, and the ambition to achieve them. They give us the incentive we need to fully participate in the play of life and to reach towards our potential as human beings. Over the years, many people have willingly shared with me their creative ideas and expressed an eagerness to achieve their goals, or to bring their ideas into physical reality. In our conversations, people will often say, "This is what I want to achieve with my life ...

there must be a way for me to do it ... look at what so and so has done!" Or, they will say, "This is what I wish to achieve ... if only there weren't certain obstacles in my path." This brings me to certain observations I would like to share.

There are many people who are very good at forming ideas, or articulating these ideas as words and sharing them with others. This makes for excellent conversation over coffee or tea. The creative impulse runs strong with these people in the emotional and mental realms, yet they seem unable to take the necessary steps to bring their ideas into reality. The words flow with gusto; but those words are the same year after year. Likewise, there are persons who have excellent ideas, but are prone to perceiving only obstacles to their realization. Granted, in some cases, the obstacles may actually exist, but, as in the first example above, there doesn't seem to be a prolonged effort to overcome them.

The point I wish to emphasize here is that if you have a goal that you very much want to achieve, there must be a concerted and prolonged effort to achieve it. If the goal is important enough to you, then it must become your focus—something to which you are willing to devote much energy over the long haul. Too many people make the mistake of wishing for something today and forgetting about it tomorrow, or until the next coffee session at the local restaurant, where the creative juices flow freely again. It takes persistence to achieve something truly worthwhile. As the Buddha is reputed to have said: "When you fix your heart on one point then nothing is impossible for you."

Let me give a personal example to illustrate the importance of concentrated focus and persistence in reaching one's goals. In 1993, I completed *Micmac Medicines: Remedies and Recollections*. This book has sold very well since its release, and

I have met many wonderful people because of its publication. However, the book was not easy, requiring much dedicated effort and time to complete. There are many professional journalists who can sit at a typewriter or word processor and complete a chapter at a single sitting. I'm not able to work that fast. When I wrote that book, my focus was very good, as hardly a day passed that I didn't write a paragraph or a page, do a line drawing, or rewrite a portion of the text. I would carry my notebook wherever I went, making notes at the beach, by the lakeshore, in the woods, at shopping malls, and in restaurants. I worked hard mentally and physically to write that book; this hard work was accompanied by work on the emotional and spiritual levels—creatively visualizing the finished product.

To reach a goal, there must be a willingness to sacrifice other things of lesser importance. As a naturalist, I'm faced with this situation quite often. I like to spend as much time as possible at outdoor activities, but often find that I'm spending a disproportionate amount of time in my car or in town. I have to stop myself and say, "Wait a minute, what's happening here? I gain a lot of my inspiration when I am in the forest, or walking the shoreline of a lake, but I'm not doing that lately." Then I try to reorganize my affairs and set priorities. This is sometimes a difficult thing for me to do, as I get stuck in my routine very easily.

III

IT IS important to visualize our goal or product as already complete or accomplished. Then we should work persistently on the physical level to help the goal manifest there. Don't make the mistake of thinking that visualization is enough, and that if properly performed the desired goal will fall from the sky into your lap! Unfortunately, this isn't going to happen. Rather, what you may find happening as a result of your visualization is that obstacles are more easily overcome, that pieces of the puzzle fall easily into place, unexpectedly bringing the goal within your grasp. Paramahansa Yogananda explained the necessity of acting on your goals with the comment, "When you make up your mind to do good things, you will accomplish them if you use dynamic will power to follow through" (Yogananda, p. 430).

This is part of the secret to prosperity. I am not speaking of prosperity from the purely financial point of view. There is a much larger definition of prosperity. Probably the most prosperous person is someone with excellent health, a balanced spiritual perspective on life, and a loving, joyful living in the moment. However, even when considering prosperity only from a financial point of view, the process of creative visualization is an important tool for success.

The forests, rivers, streams, or lakes are important places to seek out whenever we need time for visualization and quiet contemplation. For instance, the meditative sound of flowing water or the peaceful atmosphere of a calm, secluded cove are wonderful environments when we need to contemplate problems or important decisions in our lives. With this in mind, undertake the following exercise.

Exercise 17: Personal Growth Analysis

Choose a quiet, private, outdoor location for this exercise. Focus your attention on a primary characteristic of that location. For instance, should you choose to do the exercise in an area of tall pine trees when a breeze is blowing, you may be attracted to the sound of the wind as it whistles through the pine needles. The sound would be a primary characteristic of the place on that given day, and something on which to focus your attention. Use this focused attention to calm your mind. With calmness of mind, define what you would consider the three greatest limitations in your life. Then list three of your strong points or primary advantages in life. Finally, consider the goals you wish to achieve in the future. You may wish to make copies of the forms given below and perform the exercise often over the coming months or years.

Limitations

a) What do you consider the three greatest limitations in your life?

1.

2.

3.

b) Select one of those limitations to focus on during the coming month, and outline a strategy to minimize or eliminate its adverse effects.

Advantages
   a) What do you consider the three greatest advantages in your life?
   1.

   2.

   3.

   b) Select one of those advantages to focus on during the coming month and outline a strategy to maximize its influence in your life.

Growth Goals
   a)   List three primary goals in your life.
   1.

   2.

   3.

   b) What are the steps necessary to achieve the first goal?

   c) What are the steps necessary to achieve the second goal?

d) What are the steps necessary to achieve the third goal?

e) Select one primary goal to focus on during the coming month.

The following is a series of exercises and suggestions written to encourage personal growth and goal achievement. Perform exercises 20 and 21 on a regular basis, several times a week. Also, continue to use the Transformation Affirmation, making it a regular part of your daily activities.

Exercise *18*: *Exploring a New Landscape*

This exercise requires that you know how to use a compass. It should be performed only when you are accompanied by a companion.

You and your companion should go to a forested location unfamiliar to you but familiar to your companion, in case you require assistance. Using the compass as a guide, walk directly into the forest for a period of 10 to 20 minutes. Your companion should remain at the departure point, within shouting distance (have a verbal exchange every few minutes to ensure communication). When you have walked for at least ten minutes, stop, examine the landscape, and familiarize yourself with that location. You have pushed yourself into unknown territory, and have the ability to do the same in other areas of life, or with subjects you might have wanted to explore in the past but were not ready to try. In addition, in doing this exercise, you have demonstrated the will and determination to overcome your limitations.

Mentally affirm that you are going to explore your life goals with the same sense of daring and adventure.

Exercise *19*: *The Group Approach*

Take steps to organize a nature therapy group in your community. You will be surprised at the number of people who are interested in using the outdoor environment for its therapeutic advantages. There are many people who will enjoy doing group work with the exercises in this book. Have the group meet once or twice a month and encourage individual members to develop their own nature-based exercises that the whole group can explore and enjoy. In general, people who hike, camp, canoe, and do other outdoor activities are taking advantage of the therapeutic value of nature without necessarily thinking about it. Perhaps this is the ideal approach; that is, to do things out of the enjoyment and pleasure you derive from them. A myriad of health benefits will flow naturally from this approach. Make it fun and informal: avoid unnecessary rules and regulations.

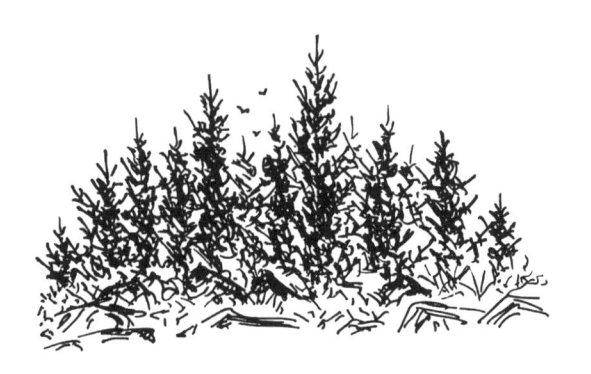

Exercise 20: Visualize Your Goal

In this exercise you are to visit your special place, taking with you a blanket, air mattress, or lawn chair on which to recline. If you are not used to lying without a pillow under your head, you will want to bring one along. It is important to be comfortable during the exercise.

At first you may wish to perform the tobacco ritual given earlier in the book. Next, find a good location to place your blanket or reclining chair. Then, sitting or standing, take several deep breaths—breathe slowly in an easy, relaxed manner. When you have completed the deep breathing, recline and make yourself comfortable. Close your eyes and, beginning with your feet, relax each part of your body. When you are fully relaxed, begin to visualize your goal on the screen of your consciousness. Visualize the goal as complete and accomplished. Take as much time as you wish, slowly building a detailed picture of your goal. When you have a complete picture of your goal, hold the image and mentally say, "It is complete!" As soon as you say those words, release the picture and forget about it. Do not dwell on it, but let it slip into the subconscious mind. Open your eyes and, beginning with the feet, slowly move each part of your body; then rise from the reclining position, and enjoy your day.

Exercise 21: The Circle Affirmation

> *The eye is the first circle; the horizon which it forms*
> *is the second; and throughout nature this*
> *primary picture is repeated without end.*
> *It is the highest emblem in the cipher of the world.*
>   Ralph Waldo Emerson,
>   *Essays on Spiritual Laws and Circles,* p. 38

Choose a goal you would like to accomplish, and create an affirmation for that goal. The affirmation should not exceed 15 to 20 words. Take your time while you think about each word of the affirmation, making it as meaningful as possible. When you have completed the affirmation, you should proceed to your special place, or a location that affords complete privacy. Slowly walk in a clockwise circle, carefully saying the affirmation out loud. Think and focus on the words as you say them—otherwise they will be meaningless. Continue to walk the circle, repeating the affirmation, but gradually decreasing the volume of your speech until the affirmation becomes a silent mental repetition. At this point, continue to walk the circle, silently repeating the words until you are satisfied that you have expressed the full meaning and depth of the affirmation. Finally, stop and take a deep breath; as you exhale, release the affirmation from your mind and leave the circle.

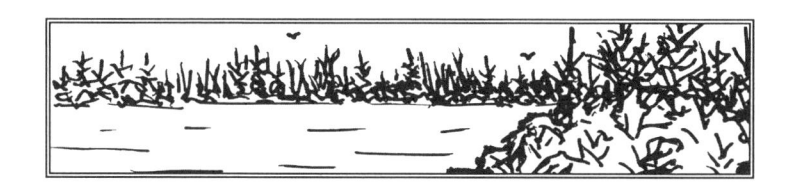

Chapter 6

EXPLORING MEDITATION

> *Place yourself in the middle of the stream of power and wisdom which flows into your life, place yourself in the full center of that flood, then you are without effort impelled to truth, to right and a perfect contentment.*
>
> Ralph Waldo Emerson,
> Essays on Spiritual Laws and Cycles, pp. 12-13

MEDITATION can play an important role in our lives, and one need not be a religious person or even someone with a spiritual philosophy to benefit from its practice. Many books about meditation approach the practice from a religious perspective. But while meditation can be the vehicle to profound spiritual and religious experience and, from my point of view, is absolutely necessary on the spiritual path, it is not necessary to discuss meditation strictly from a spiritual or religious point of view.

What are we to make of this apparent paradox? Why should an atheist be able to benefit from meditation—a practice religious and spiritually minded people have cherished as their own and guarded for centuries? To approach this question we should consider meditation as a "vehicle." For instance, an automobile is analogous to meditation in that it will transport a person from point A to point B, as long as the person knows how to drive and follows the rules of the road. Similarly, if you know the process of meditation, and follow the guidelines provided by others experienced in the practice, your body and mind will respond appropriately, whether you are a saintly person or a money-hungry capitalist. The techniques and processes of meditation are impersonal. Benefits to the body and mind will always follow, if an individual practices a valid, time-proven form of meditation. Of course, the greatest benefits are achieved by those who practise regularly over a long period of time. The following list of some of the benefits of meditation illustrates the marvellous results you may experience through regular practice.

1. Meditation lowers and helps to control high blood pressure. The calming influence of meditation is probably the reason for its effects on blood pressure. People with high blood pressure should not abandon their medication when they begin meditating. Although you may find that your blood pressure improves significantly, your doctor should monitor your blood pressure regularly and advise you regarding any adjustment of your medication.

2. Meditation helps reduce stress. Just as meditation is beneficial to people with high blood pressure, it is also a natural way to relieve stress and its adverse effects. Again, its effectiveness in reducing stress is probably due to its relaxing and calming influence on the mind.

3. Meditation leads to improved performance and greater self-confidence. Individuals who meditate regularly may notice an improvement in committing things to memory and in memory recall. Others report having more energy, an increased ability to concentrate, and improved self-esteem. Clearly the confidence factor is important, and it's one of the benefits I notice most when I meditate regularly.

4. *Meditation promotes a balanced approach to life.* The practice of meditation tends to improve one's outlook on life, filling the world with fresh, positive potential. Meditation leads to a positive anticipation and a creative attitude towards each new moment of our lives.

5. *There is a feeling of joy in meditation.* With continuous practice, this joy is carried beyond the meditative state into daily life as a lasting, joyful state of mind.

> *If, when there is quiet, the spirit has*
> *continuously and uninterruptedly a sense of*
> *great joy as if intoxicated or freshly bathed,*
> *it is a sign that the light-principle is*
> *harmonious in the whole body; then the Golden*
> *Flower begins to bud.*
>
> The Secret of the Golden Flower:
A Chinese Book of Life, p. 49

Those not familiar with meditation often ask about the relationship between concentration and meditation. To some extent the difference is intellectual rather than practical, in that it has little bearing on our practice. For the purposes of the exercises in this book, it is not necessary to differentiate between the two states of mind. However, readers who delve deeper into the subject of meditation will certainly become aware that yoga masters and other adepts do differeniate carefully between concentration and meditation. Some define meditation as concentration focussed on the Divine or on

Divine manifestations. To concentrate or focus on Divine Love, for instance, is meditation. If, during our meditation, we feel as if we are bathed in this Love, we have achieved a deep meditative state. Similarly, to achieve a state of peace and calmness of mind is also meditation. Meditation is experiencing and maintaining serenely a particular state of mind that brings one in relationship with spirit.

On the other hand, to focus on images or on external things—such as a flower, candle, or some other object—is concentration. Concentration is a preparation for meditation; a prelude to the contemplative state.

*Meditation ... is only the sustained attitude
of the concentrated mind in face of an object
of devotion, or a problem that needs illumination
to be intelligible, of anything whereof the life
is to be realised and absorbed, rather than the
form.*

Annie Besant
Thought Power, Its Control and Practice, p. 105

Meditation requires privacy and solitude. It is possible, however, to meditate almost any place, even in a crowded shopping mall! But unless we are highly skilled in the practice, such public meditation will be shallow at best, since our attention will not be focused. It is much easier to focus, or to attain a calmness of mind, when you know that you have complete privacy. Group meditation is beneficial as well. In some respects it has the potential to be more powerful and helpful than solitary practice. The atmosphere created by group meditation supports one's efforts and inspires a person to practise regularly. It must be stressed that the best results are always achieved through regular meditation, as daily meditation has cumulative effects. Of course, if you find it is impossible to meditate regularly, even a little meditation is better than none. It is also helpful to meditate in the same location. When we become familiar with a place, meditation is easier, partly because the mind associates the location with the practice. By continuing to meditate in the same place, you create vibrations conducive to the practice of meditation.

Don't allow yourself to become frustrated if your practice isn't going as well as you think it should. Frustration must be avoided like a plague! When your mind wanders during meditation, accept this as part of the learning experience, and don't allow it to ruin the good effects you might have experienced. Many people try too hard and have all kinds of unrealistic expectations. The important thing is to keep practising, regardless of how much your mind wanders, and to bring it back to whatever you were concentrating on, or to re-assume the state of meditative calmness whenever you notice that you have lost attention. Many who have read and studied spiritual, psychic, occult, or New Age literature, worry about negative influences affecting their mind, aura, chakras, or energy fields during concentration and meditation practices. These people often counter such fear by mentally visualizing themselves surrounded by White Light during their practice. If you have followed this procedure in the past, continue to do so while practising the exercises suggested below.

Personally, I have always felt that the fear of such negative influence is overstated, and assumes more importance than it deserves. Over the twenty-five years that I have been a student of metaphysical and mystical philosophy, I have tried many practices, but have never felt the need to protect myself in this way. Periodically I have practised the White

Light visualization as an energy exercise, but have never used it for protective purposes. In my view, the human being is not a puppet at the mercy of any negative influence that might happen its way. Rather, we have our own involuntary protective force, which is the Self, the Inner Guardian of the human temple, ever alert (even while we sleep), and which I have never seen the need to reinforce during my meditative practices. Indeed, all forms of concentration and mediation in which the mind is active in a virtuous and positive way, are perfectly safe.

If you wish to reach deep states of meditative awareness you must also consider your posture. Without good posture, it is difficult to relax, as tensions in the body prevent successful meditative practice. Your spine should be straight, which is probably the most important part of correct posture, as otherwise you will not derive maximum benefit from the energy flow in your spine during meditation. However, I am not suggesting the use of traditional yogic postures, even though if you can comfortably assume those positions, they are most useful. Many people have difficulty assuming certain postures, which creates frustration. A person may become so uncomfortable in his or her attempt to assume a particular position, that the posture loses any value it might have had! There is only one rule you should follow: keep your spine as straight as possible and assume a position that you can hold comfortably for a prolonged period of time. The important thing is to relax and to be comfortable. If you are confined to a wheelchair, or handicapped in some other way, make yourself comfortable in your usual or familiar manner. You can still have a successful meditation, regardless of physical limitations. Nature always finds a way to compensate. In the words of a Zen Master: "If you find it impossible to sit because of some pain or some physical difficulty, then you should sit anyway, using a thick cushion or a chair. Even though you are the worst horse you will get to the marrow of Zen" (Suzuki, pp. 39-40).

There are people who can meditate in a prone position, and find it beneficial; they should continue in this manner. It is easy to fall asleep in this position, so they must guard against this happening. The main thing is to be comfortable, and to have a beneficial experience.

The relationship of nature or the natural environment to meditation has a long history. For centuries, retreats, hermitages, and monasteries have been built in isolated areas. Those locations were generally selected because they afforded privacy to commune with the Great Spirit in the natural beauty of the landscape, unaltered by the works of human kind. The ancients recognized the value of mountains, valleys, streams, lakes, and forests to the practice of concentration and meditation. The beautiful landscape was recognized as a catalyst to Divine Communion, and the realization of higher spiritual dimensions. Certain special places lent themselves to the reception of the higher vibratory forces. Centuries later, great personages such as Meister Eckhart, William Blake, Red Cloud, Black Elk, Helen Blavatsky, Walt Whitman, Richard Bucke, Henry David Thoreau, Ralph Waldo Emerson, and Paramahansa Yogananda, all recognized the importance of nature to the full expression of the human spirit.

In this age of computer technology, we need to find balance in our lives—we need to connect with our origins in the natural world. We need to rediscover the benefits of nature's landscape to the quality of our spiritual lives; how the natural world can help us to maintain health and remedy personal problems.

The following are three exercises in concentration and meditation. Try each of the exercises several times, or until you discover which exercise is most beneficial to your personality and life situation. Then practise it regularly, making it part of your daily or weekly routine.

Exercise 22: *Walking Meditation*

Select a quiet country road, a wooded path, a lake shore, or a private beach. The place you choose should have a minimum amount of interference and noise. Stand facing the direction you intend to walk. Examine the path ahead of you and the surrounding environment; try to establish a sense of harmony with your surroundings. Think positively about the meditative practice you are about to begin. Remind yourself of its importance to your life. Slowly take several deep breaths, freeing your mind of the baggage of worries or fears you may be carrying with you.

Focus attention on your feet; consider how they feel against the ground. Begin to walk at a slow, even pace. Pay attention to your steps in the same way you learned to attend to the rhythm of your breathing in an earlier exercise on concentration. Do not strain your mind, relax your forehead, and walk slowly, easily, and purposefully. Follow your footsteps—first the left, then the right, then the left, and so on. Notice the even rhythm of your steps, and the texture of the ground as first your left foot, then your right foot, continuously touch the earth. Try to sense a harmony or a relationship with the earth. Allow your mind to meditate on this connection to the earth mother. Notice the calm state of your mind. Enjoy this state as you continue walking for several minutes. Finally, come to a stop, stand still with closed eyes, and relax within the serenity of your mind. After a few minutes, open your eyes, completing the meditation.

Exercise 23: The Beauty and Joy Meditation

This exercise should be done in a setting that is both beautiful and peaceful. It should offer the privacy you need during meditation. If you wish, perform this exercise in your special place.

Assume a comfortable posture, and take three deep breaths, inhaling and exhaling slowly. Calmly survey the landscape with your eyes—consider the beauty you find there, and how much it means to you. Think of the difference beauty makes to life, and how drab the world would be without it. Resolve in the future to take the time to fully appreciate the beauty in your life. Consider whether the outward beauty you see in the landscape is the same as the inner beauty you meet in people. Spend several minutes contemplating this question.

Continue to examine the landscape, thinking about the importance of joy to life. You can find beauty in the landscape. Can you find joy as well? Both of these qualities are intangibles, yet when we look at a sunset we can find beauty and joy. Contemplate the relationship between beauty and joy as you examine the landscape in front of you.

After several minutes, close your eyes, and attempt to feel joy. Focus on the pit of your stomach, and try to feel joy at that point (it may come as a "ticklish" feeling in your stomach). Gradually allow it to spread through your entire body;

feel the joy everywhere. Remain relaxed, and feel it expand beyond your body, spreading out over the landscape around you. Allow yourself to meditate on the impressions of joy, maintaining the vibrations. Complete the meditation at your own pace.

Exercise 24: The Earth Meditation

This meditation may be done at any location offering privacy. This is a meditation in which you assert your affinity for the earth, so I suggest you do it in your special place.

Relax, assume a comfortable posture, and take several deep breaths. Close your eyes. Feel the earth beneath you. Take a few minutes to think about the earth, its position in the solar system, and in the greater universe. Think about yourself and the importance of the earth to your life. Again, focus on the earth beneath you; imagine a stream of energy coming from the earth, moving up into your body, and following the spine to your head and beyond. Calmly meditate on that energy and on the feeling of connectedness to the earth.

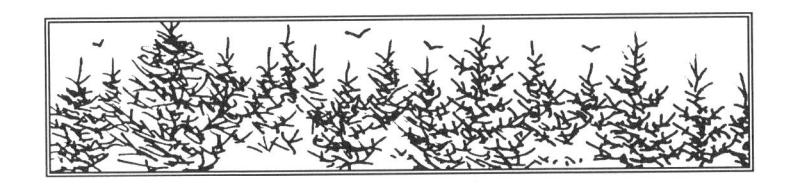

Chapter 7

DISCOVERING THE WILD EDIBLES

THERE is a great deal of enjoyment and satisfaction in exploring the forests and fields for wild edibles. One derives a certain pleasure in harvesting wild foods, partly because they are free and usually not available at supermarkets. This is especially true of berries, if you happen to live in an area where they are plentiful. The wild blueberry is a good example. I often go into the field in late July and August to pick large bowls full of these berries. This practice is very gratifying and therapeutic. While picking blueberries I usually enjoy a peaceful, meditative state. In fact, a field of blueberries is like a giant mother earth rosary—picking berries is much like saying the rosary as a meditative practice. Lately I've been eating blueberries fresh off the bush, as a summer tonic. I got the idea from a raven that spends much of its time in my field during berry season. I decided to follow his lead, and now sit in the field, enjoying the blueberries by the handfuls, on summer evenings.

Of course, not everyone has the luxury of picking berries. I was fortunate to be born a free berry picker—my parents owned property on which berries grew. The availability of berries continues to the present day. However, even if you have to pay to pick your berries, it is still very satisfying; just knowing that you can make something delicious with them is reward enough. This is nature therapy at its best.

Wild teas are also very enjoyable. Mints, labrador tea, sweet fern, witch hazel, and strawberry, among others, are interesting plants with which to experiment. The primary benefit of searching for wild edibles, from a therapeutic perspective, is to be able to locate and enjoy the occasional sampling of wild foods. I have never especially enjoyed wild treats made from roots, leaves, and bark. There are several that I like, but the remainder I would eat only in an emergency. The potential of wild plants as a food source in survival situations is the chief reason we should learn to identify the plants and trees that can be relied upon to provide nourishment for the body. However, it is important to stress that plants may become endangered if over-harvested in a given area. One should harvest wild edibles only occasionally, or in emergency situations. If you harvest plants faster than they can reproduce, you will have a detrimental impact on the local ecosystem.

Some people think you cannot cause serious ecological damage by the extensive harvesting of plants that have been introduced into a new landscape. While this may be true, I have reservations about it. Any plant that has become established in a given environment must be approached with respect. For example, many introduced plants add immensely to the richness of our environment. If we were to attempt to eradicate or over-collect plantain and mustards, for instance, it would be a terrible shame from a medicinal perspective. These are wonderful medicine plants, and it is a joy to find them growing in North America. Or, for instance, consider the beauty of the dandelion. I cannot imagine going through a spring season without the striking colour and wonderful mild perfume of that plant.

As we gain an appreciation for the value of plant life, or become increasingly aware of the benefits the natural environment offers us, we become more sensitive to the way we interact with the environment and the life forms in it. This is a new awakening for each of us personally; a realization that we do make a difference. We may not be able to control the actions of society at large—and the way individuals interact with the earth, its life forms, and resources—but we do have much control over our own actions and our way of life. Our lives can set positive examples to others, if we live in a way that reflects our sensitivity and enjoyment of nature.

This new awakening may inspire you to study the value and benefits of even those plants most commonly designated as garden weeds. You may learn to cherish those so-called weeds as much as you cherish your most valuable ornamental plant or garden vegetable. When you collect plants as medicines or foods, you will do so with the plant uppermost in mind, always careful that you do not endanger its existence in a given location, and always thankful for the gifts it gives to you. I believe this is the ethical approach towards plant life and our mother earth.

THE WILD FOODS AND TEAS

What follows is a selection of wild treats to tempt your taste buds and test your identification skills. Bear in mind that the taste of a species may vary from place to place, depending on its genetic properties and the composition of the soil—or substances that may have been added to the soil by humans or other animals (Elias, p. 9). Also, for identification purposes, it is advisable to use several plant manuals on your field excursions. Remember, when foraging for edibles, always be absolutely certain you have correctly identified each plant. This is particularly true for mushrooms, as there are only minor differences between certain poisonous and non-poisonous species.

Arrowhead, Common, *Sagittaria latifolia* Willd

This plant grows around the margins of lakes, in ponds, streams, swamps, and generally where there is shallow water. The fruit and tuberous roots are good as food, although they may have a bitter taste if eaten raw. They are best harvested in late summer through to early spring. You may need a digging stick to collect them, as you have to loosen the roots from the muddy bottom where they grow. The tubers float to the surface and are easily collected. The tubers may be roasted, baked, or boiled like a potato. Boil for approximately 30 minutes, or until tender, and then peel and serve with butter.

Arrowhead

Bayberry, *Myrica pensylvanica* Loisel

This plant is generally very easy to locate. It grows near swamps, around the margin of ponds and lakes, and on old fields, alongside blueberry and sweet fern. The leaves can be used as a spice, or brewed to make a tea. You can pick the leaves anytime, but they are probably most aromatic in July and August. After picking, wash and allow them to dry thoroughly in a warm, shaded area. They should be spread out over a large surface for this purpose. Store the leaves in a tightly sealed jar away from the light (e.g., in a dark cupboard).

Bayberry leaves can be crushed and used in stews, sauces, and on meat or fish. As a tea, use approximately one tablespoon of bayberry leaves for one and a half cups of water, steeping for ten minutes.

Bayberry

Bearberry, *Arctosphylos Uva-ursi* (L.) Spreng

The bearberry plant grows on rocky or sandy soils in many areas of North America. It produces nutritious—though rather bland and astringent—berries. However, their taste is improved if they are stewed with sugar and eaten with cream. These berries are valuable as a survival food source. The leaves are smoked by Native peoples as a substitute for tobacco (*Nicotiana*). The bearberry is often referred to as *kinnickinnick*, although this term rightly applies to a tobacco-like mixture made from several plants of which the bearberry is just one.

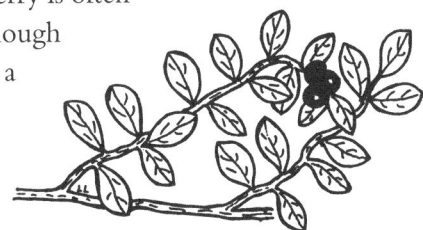

Bearberry

67

Beech, *Fagus grandifolia* Ehrh
This tree is very common in eastern Canada and the eastern United States. It grows in large stands, or in mixed forests. The nuts may be gathered when they fall after a heavy frost. You can separate the burrs from the nuts individually, or by shaking them. They should be dried in an open, warm area. The nuts may be cracked by heating them in an oven, which makes it easier to remove the shells. They are edible raw, ground into flour, or roasted and ground as a coffee substitute. You can also extract a cooking oil from the nuts by crushing them and boiling them in water, and then skimming the oil from the surface.

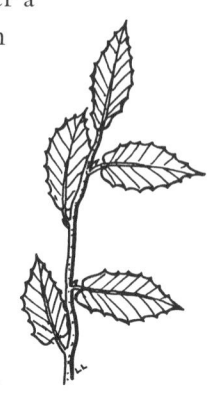

Beech

Birch, Yellow, *Betula alleghaniensis* Britt
The birch trees are valuable for many reasons. They have food value and yield a variety of products. For example, you can make a medicinal tea from yellow birch bark, or use the sap from white birch bark as a tonic. It can be boiled down, like maple sap, to make syrup or sugar. Tap the sap as you would sugar maple, but do it a few weeks later in the springtime. The ratio of sap to syrup is far greater than for maple trees. When tapping birch, be careful to plug the tree well, as it can be difficult to stop the flow of sap, which could possibly kill the tree. The inner bark of yellow birch can be eaten raw or boiled as survival food. The bark may be dried and ground into flour. For tea, steep the leaves or inner bark in water or, with white birch, especially in the birch sap.

Yellow birch

Burdock, *Arctium minus* (Hill) Bernh

The burdock is a strong medicine plant, especially as a blood tonic against skin rashes and other skin problems caused by impurities in the blood. The roots are very beneficial in this respect. Aside from its medicinal benefits, burdock is useful as a food source. The young first-year roots are best, and may be harvested during the summer. To prepare, peel, slice, and boil the roots in water. In *Edible Wild Plants, a North American Field Guide*, Elias and Dykeman mention adding a pinch of baking soda to the water and boiling for 20 minutes; they also suggest changing the water after that time and boiling the roots until tender (p. 112). You can then serve the burdock root with butter, or whatever meets your fancy. The first-year basal leaf stalks and second-year flower stalks may also be peeled and eaten, either cooked or in salads.

Burdock

Cattail, Broad Leaf, *Typha latifolia* L.

The cattail grows in swamps, shallow ponds, and other wet areas, such as along the edge of streams. It is a well-known edible and a good emergency food. The sprouts at the end of the roots are good to eat in early spring, either raw or cooked. Later in the season, sprouts appear on the roots at the base of the leaves. Pull the leafy stalks by grasping them below the water surface (they often break off at the roots), then peel away the outer layers to reveal the tender core, which can be eaten raw or cooked. The green bloom spikes are also edible. They should be picked before the pollen ripens above

Cattails

them, and while still in their papery sheaths. To prepare for eating, the sheaths must be removed and the spikes boiled in salted water until tender. The buds may then be plucked from the core of the spike and eaten. Both the pollen and the core of the root may be substituted for regular flour. The pollen can be collected and added to a recipe using flour. The root core should be crushed, the fibers strained, and the remaining starch washed several times. (See Elias and Dykeman, p. 69.) This can be dried, or used wet. The root core may also be cooked in salted water and eaten as a vegetable. (The narrow leaf cattail, *Typha angustifolia* L., may be used similarly.)

Crowberry, *Empetrum nigrum* L.

You can find crowberry plants in bogs, in such open places as acid barrens, or on cliffs near the ocean. They are excellent ground cover, preventing erosion. The berries are recommended as a survival food. They are especially good as emergency food because they are very juicy and will quench the thirst. Also, since the plant is an evergreen, the berries are available all year, which certainly enhances their value. The crowberry's reputation as a taste-treat varies somewhat—one author states that they have "a very faint, pleasant taste." Another writes that the enjoyment of the berries is "an acquired taste." I find crowberries pleasant, but not something I would crave, such as blueberries. Apparently, cooking the berries with the addition of sugar and lemon improves their palatability. I've always enjoyed finding crowberries, and sampling them as a wild treat.

Crowberry

Dandelion, *Taraxacum officinale* Weber

The dandelion is amazing for its rich vitamin and mineral content. The plant was introduced from Europe, and is found growing on fields, lawns, old farmlands, and other uncultivated areas. It is a valuable food plant. The young leaves can be used in salads or cooked as greens if they are gathered before they flower and become bitter. The roots can be cooked in the same fashion as carrots, or they can be roasted slowly, ground into a powder, and used as a coffee substitute. For cooking purposes, the roots can be dug from the time the leaves first appear, until they become bitter. As a substitute for coffee, dig the roots in autumn. The yellow petals from the dandelion make an excellent wine, and many wine-making books offer recipes extolling their virtues.

Dandelion

Jewelweed, *Impatiens capensis* Meerb, and *Impatiens pallida* Nutt

The jewelweed is also termed "Touch-Me-Not," and is found growing near wet places such as ditches or brooks. It has many uses as a medicine plant, including using its juices to relieve the itch of poison ivy blisters. As a food plant, the young shoots may be boiled in water for 15 minutes, drained and washed twice more in boiling water, then seasoned before eating. A note of caution: because the plant contains calcium oxalate crystals, it should only be used infrequently as a food plant. However, prepared as described above, it is safe as an emergency food. The ripe seeds may be separated from their pods and eaten as an emergency food source.

Jewelweed

Lettuce, Wild, *Lactuca canadensis* L., and many other varieties

The wild lettuce often grows in wet places and cut-over areas. The leaves should be picked and eaten while the plant is still young and less than four to six inches tall. They can be eaten on their own or used with other greens in a tossed salad. Some people boil the leaves in a small amount of water for a few minutes, and serve them with seasonings. A note of caution: the leaves should be eaten sparingly, since when eaten raw, in large quantities, they may cause digestive problems.

Wild lettuce

Mountain Ash, *Sorbus americana* Marsh

The fruit of this tree may be eaten during the fall and winter months—if you can beat the birds to them! In fact, some people feel the berries become more palatable after a couple of frosts, when they are also more easily plucked from the twigs. The fruit is certainly a good emergency food source. They may be prepared in a manner similar to cranberries, and used for the same purposes.

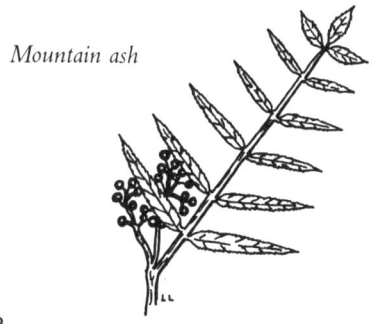

Mountain ash

Nettle, Stinging, *Urtica dioica* L.

This plant is found growing along roads, trails, and stream banks. As its name implies, it is covered with stiff, stinging hairs. Because of this, one should wear gloves when harvesting the plant. To destroy the irritant, barely cover the plants in water and boil for one minute, and then simmer until tender. Drain the water, and season to taste. The stinging nettle is high in protein, minerals, and vitamins A and C.

Stinging nettle

Oak, Red, *Quercus borealis* Michx. f., and other varieties

The red oak likes to grow in well-drained soils, and is often found growing in valleys as well as on slopes of hills. The acorns can be gathered in autumn as they fall from the trees. They should be stored in a cool, dry place. Of course, the acorns may also be shelled and eaten immediately after gathering. However, the bitterness must be removed from the meat. Boil the shelled nuts in water until the water turns brown, then repeat the process several times until the water remains clear. Alternatively, the shelled nuts may be placed in running water, such as a brook, until their bitterness is washed away. This may take a day or more to accomplish.

Red oak

Peppermint, *Mentha piperita* L.

    A primary characteristic of mints is that they have four-sided (square-edged) stems. This feature, combined with their fragrant leaves, make them relatively easy to identify. Peppermint leaves have a distinct smell when broken or crushed; peppermint may also be identified by its purple stem. It grows in wet meadows and along streams.

    The leaves may be picked at any stage of growth, and dried in a warm place. However, they can be used either dried or fresh. Peppermint can be used in tea, salads, or in sweet dishes.

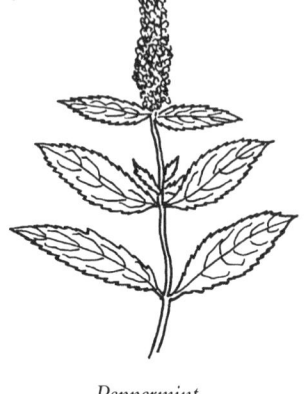

Peppermint

Pickerel Weed, *Pontederia cordata* L.

    This plant grows in mucky areas along the margins of lakes, ponds, and slow-moving streams. Its beautiful blue flowers stand proudly above the water, making it easy to identify in summer. The seeds are edible and should be collected from the mature spikes. Edible fresh, they can also be dried and added to baked goods, such as breads. The young leafstalks, picked in early summer, can be eaten as salad.

Pickerel weed

Rose, Common Wild, *Rosa virginiana* Mill, R. *carolina* Marsh, and others

Wild roses grow in pastures, roadsides, and along the heads of salt marshes, among other areas. The petals can be nibbled as a sweet treat, or used to make wine. (I find, however, that the wine resembles perfume!) The rosehips can be used to make jam, or dried and used for tea. They are rich in vitamin C, and also contain beta-carotene as well as vitamins E, B, and K. There are many interesting uses for roses, including medicinal ones: for instance, some Native peoples used the roots and leaves in a spring tonic preparation. The roots are also used to treat diarrhea.

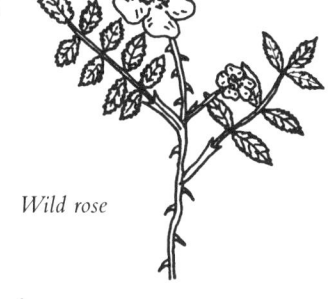

Wild rose

Sweet Fern, *Comptonia peregrina* (L.) Coult

The sweet fern grows near the edge of fields, along roadsides, and in barren areas. The leaves may be used to make a pleasant-tasting tea. Prepare as directed in the medicinal plant index. The young nutlets may be eaten as food. They should be gathered in June and July.

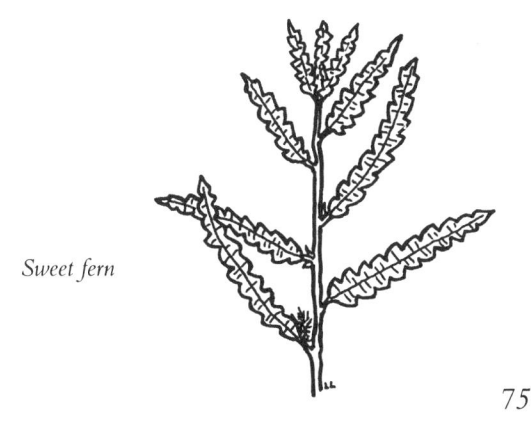

Sweet fern

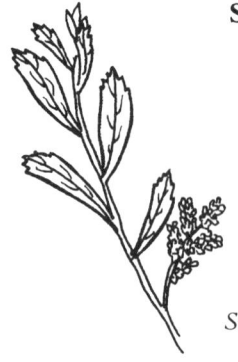

Sweet Gale, *Myrica gale* L.

This plant grows around the margins of lakes, streams, and swamps. The uses for sweet gale are similar to those for bayberry. Its nutlets can be picked and eaten raw.

Sweet Gale

Wood Sorrel, *Oxalis montana* Raf.

This plant is commonly found in damp areas, such as along mossy banks of streams, and in swamps. The sorrels have somewhat sour-tasting leaves, with a sweet accent. The wood sorrel and yellow wood sorrel (*Oxalis stricta* L.) are among my personal favourites. Wood sorrels are not related to the sorrels and docks of the genus *Rumex* L, although they have a similar flavour. Both sorrels are best enjoyed raw.

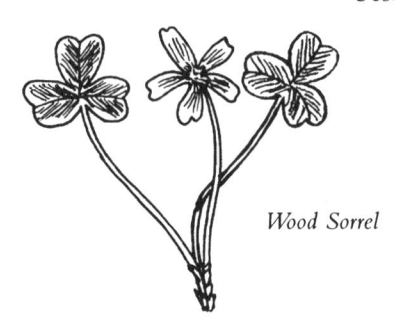

Wood Sorrel

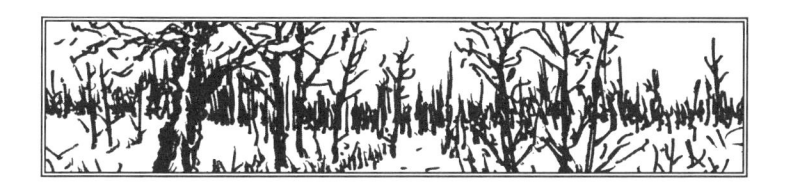

Chapter 8

MEDICINE WALK

THE notion of a "medicine walk" conveys the impression of walking the forest for the purpose of discovering or learning about the medicinal nature of plants and trees, and their many uses in human society. However, as used in this book, the concept has a much broader, wide-ranging connotation and meaning. A medicine walk is healing in its own right, and has a spiritual dimension. It is healing in that participants are encouraged to leave behind their cares and worries, focusing entirely on the walk and the beauty of the natural world around them. It is also a method of fostering closer ties to the landscape, of reconnecting to mother earth. To feel deeply that we are sisters and brothers of the earth, and that we are kin to the other life forms around us, is a valuable spiritual experience and awakening. So, from my perspective, the medicine walk involves the whole person—physically, mentally, and spiritually. Everyone should feel relaxed and free to express themselves during a medicine walk: to talk, cry, sing, and laugh. They should approach a medicine walk with sincerity and open minds, welcoming experiences that may happen during the course of the walk.

I will describe this medicine walk as if it were actually happening. The walk will focus largely on the identification and use of plants in Native medicines, although other issues will be discussed. I have had many interesting experiences over the past 25 years of field walks, and will incorporate some of these into the following pages.

The weather in June can be very unpredictable in Nova Scotia. It can be as hot and dry as late July or, conversely, as damp and wet as early May. Also, the black flies and mosquitoes can be so thick as to make hiking a miserable experience. Fortunately, we have chosen a very good day, with the temperature hovering around 20° Celsius, and a clear sky, except for a few clouds drifting across the horizon to the southwest. We are in the barrens, west of Bridgewater. Earlier, in preparation for the walk, each person went to a private location to free their thoughts as much as possible of expectations, worries, or concerns. Now, as we come together to begin our hike, I take the opportunity to say a few words to the group.

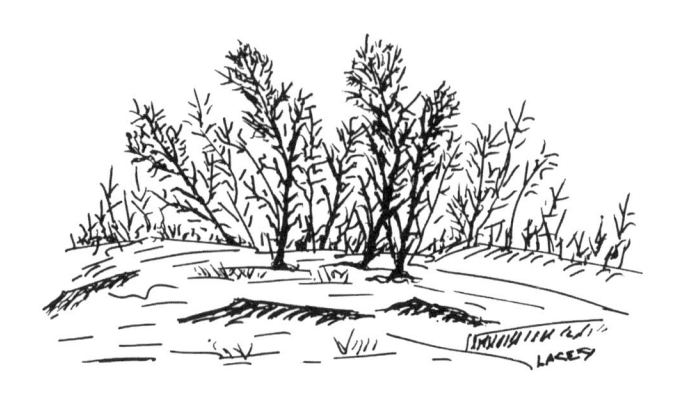

"Time is of little importance in a medicine walk. The walk may last for an hour, or it may go on for several hours, or an entire day, for that matter, depending on the circumstances. This particular walk will go for an afternoon, taking us through a variety of landscapes and learning experiences." I continue, stressing that human use of plant parts, tree barks, and other natural materials predates recorded history. I mention the excitement of the study, that it can occupy a lifetime, and that in its study we are forever students, and must remain open or receptive to new experiences in the natural world. I cite the lives of outstanding ethnobotanists, including Richard Shultz, who spent decades studying plants in the rain forests of South America, and who was greatly loved and respected by those whose lives he touched. The study of plant life must have defined Richard Shultz, and given him a great sense of worth in an often chaotic world.

   I lead the way over flat bedrock to a narrow trail winding through a stand of wire birch, to where the path ends, forcing us to make our way over rocks or through large clumps of lambkill and huckleberry bushes. Our progress is slow because of the density of this ground cover. Occasionally we hear the chirping of birds, or see a squirrel scurrying for cover from our presence in its environment. On another occasion, we stop to watch a raven observing us from the comfort of a fire-scarred pine tree, damaged by lightning. The raven, with a deep, low cackle, flies away to the west and the cover of poplar trees. As we continue over the rough terrain, a woman remarks that the medicine walk is an excellent "grounding" exercise. She adds that the thought-cleansing process prior to the walk allowed her to put aside distractions, and to focus solely on experiencing the Leipsigaek barrens area. It grounded her to the place. Now, while walking, she is able to concentrate on this environment, as if it were the only thing that mattered at the moment.

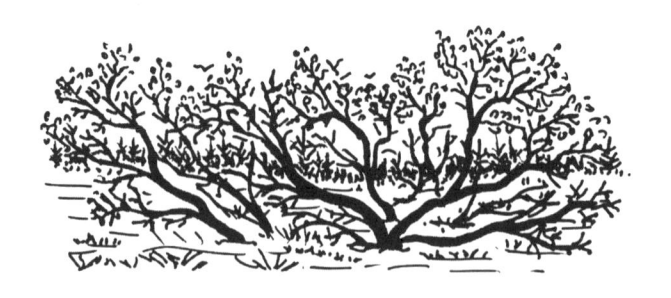

Arriving at a low, swampy area, we find a thick cover of alder bushes spreading in all directions. Many people consider alders useless shrubs, serving little or no purpose in the scheme of things. However, they are in fact excellent ground cover and, in many areas, provide a basic resource against soil erosion. Someone remarks how disconnected we have become from the natural world, and how quickly we conclude that a bush, such as the alder, is useless, without thinking about the role it plays in the environment.

I explain that for centuries the Native peoples of North America have used alder for a variety of purposes. The fresh leaves were applied to the body in poultice form to treat arthritis or sore joints. For this purpose, the leaves were heated and applied to the sore area. If the leaves became too hot, or produced a burning sensation, they were replaced with a fresh poultice of leaves. I relate that one would treat a sore wrist, for example, by placing the leaves around the wrist and keeping them in place with a bandage. It is also interesting to note that the juice from the bark, or a freshly made infusion of the bark, is used to bathe skin rashes, including poison ivy.

The dry bark and leaves of the alder were also used to treat stomach cramps. The process was very simple: the leaves and/or inner bark were steeped in water for approximately

10 minutes, and a small amount was taken internally. Green alder bark or leaves should never be taken internally; they should be dried for several days before using, to prevent cramps. The inner bark of the root, especially, has strong emetic properties.

II

WE WALK along the perimeter of the swamp, carefully observing the dense alder cover for signs of animal and bird life. Initially I had planned to move away from the swamp, but had allowed the spontaneity of the moment to change my plans. Proceeding through a particularly open area we discover a group of pitcher plants growing in a wet, mossy environment. Stepping carefully through the water-soaked moss, we examine the pitcher plants, noting that several are large, with cup-like parts measuring six to eight inches in length. I mention that as a child I was fascinated with the pitcher plant, often examining the interior of the cups for insects, and wondering about the chemical nature of the fluid they contained. I remark that the Mi'kmaq called the plant "Indian Cup Root," and that the root was used to treat tuberculosis and kidney ailments, probably including kidney stones. For this purpose, a piece of the root was steeped in water, and the liquid taken internally. It may have been taken in small dosages, perhaps half a cupful at a time. This concoction was also considered useful for indigestion.

Making our way to the far end of the swamp, we see a small, low island, rising perhaps a foot above the surface of the water-soaked spaghnum moss encircling it. There are several hackmatack trees growing on the island; they are small, but have the appearance of age, evidenced by the roughness of their bark and by their short, dry branches. Someone remarks that the hackmatack may be close to a century old. She notes that the size of these trees in this swampy environment is certainly not indicative of their longevity. I agree, and mention that a friend of mine cut a hackmatack he found growing in a bog, and determined that it was at least 70 years old.

The Mi'kmaq people used hackmatack to treat festering wounds, although there are no records as to how exactly they used it. I imagine they would have softened the inner bark, perhaps crushing it, and placing it in poultice form on the wound. Then again, it might have been made into a bathing solution for treating wounds. In Europe, hackmatack was used externally to treat eczema and psoriasis. The Mi'kmaq also use a tea made from the twigs and inner bark to treat colds and influenza. The tea is prepared by steeping one ounce of the inner bark in one pint of water for 10-15 minutes. A cup of the tea may be taken twice daily.

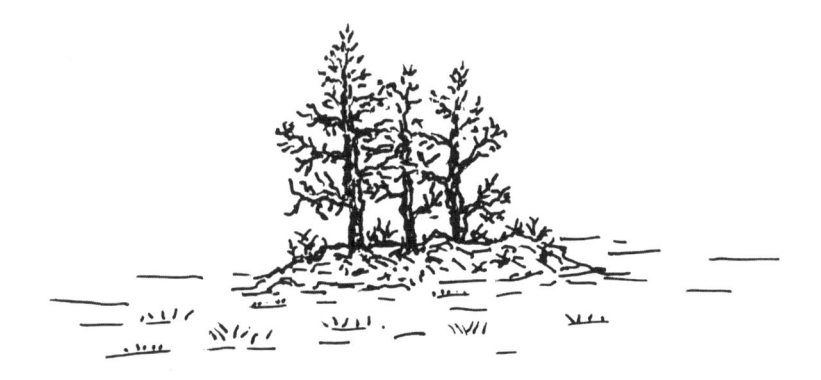

We move away from the swamp in an easterly direction towards a small knoll with a stand of white birch. The birches are brilliant white in the warm sun, with their leaves fluttering in the soft breeze. On reaching the knoll we discover it is free of the thick undergrowth that has thus far hampered our progress. In fact, we are so happy for this change in environment that we decide to tarry there, resting on the small granite boulders scattered among the birch trees.

Margaret, an artist in her early twenties, seated on the rock nearest to me, remarks that she cannot forget the hackmatacks. She adds that she would have liked to paint them using watercolours. Steven, an avid hiker, responds: "Imagine how it would be to remain in one location, like those hackmatacks, observing the same environment for 70 to 100 years! You would see the coming and going of the seasons, the changing water levels; hear the peeping of frogs in the spring, the relative quiet of winter; and experience the constant changes in the weather, and the life and death of many species as they interact with the landscape."

"Yes, what a story those old hackmatack could tell us," a third person interjects. "If we knew something about trees … I mean … if we studied those trees, I bet they would tell us a great deal; the physical characteristics of those trees must tell an interesting story—if we knew how to read it."

"Sure, even little things," Margaret replies. "You might notice a thicker growth of twigs and leaves on the south side, since it is the warm side, or that the hackmatack bend to the east or southeast, even slightly, indicative of the strong west or northwesterly winds over the years. I'm sure the bark and roots tell a story as well."

We leave that place, moving slowly towards Leipsigaek Lake. Soon we come upon a gully running north to south, replete with chunks of broken bedrock, the result of mining operations some 50 to 70 years earlier. Some of the bedrock fragments are the result of frost or other natural forces, while other pieces appear to have been broken by human hands, perhaps obsessed with the smell, texture, colour, and wealth that gold might offer to those lucky enough to find it in abundance. Following the gully we reach an area rich in medicinal plant species. I decide to stop and talk about some of the plants growing here.

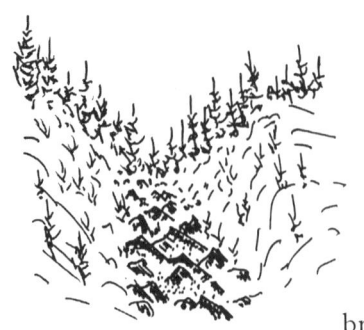

I explain that bunchberry belongs to the dogwood family of plants, as evidenced by its leaves. Several members of this family of plants were used as traditional medicines in Native cultures. Bunchberries are edible in both a raw or cooked state. In Mi'kmaq medicine, the leaves of bunchberry were applied to wounds to stop bleeding and to promote healing. The leaves were steeped and used as tea to treat kidney ailments (approximately four to six leaves to one cup of water). The Blackfoot people used the bark of a related species, red osier dogwood, to treat chest colds and liver disorders. I finish my explanation by noting that people have eaten the berries to counter the effects of poisoning. Terry Willard mentions that he used the bunchberry plant to successfully treat himself for mushroom poisoning (Willard, p. 158). I suspect that both the leaves and berries would be effective in this respect.

We walk to an area of wild sarsaparilla shoots growing deep in the gully. This plant found medicinal use in many North American Native cultures. The roots were frequently used; they were probably boiled until soft, and applied in poultice form to wounds and sores, chewed, or made into a tea to treat colds and influenza. Steep one ounce in a pint of water for ten minutes and take a cup of the tea two or three times daily. Occasionally people confuse wild sarsaparilla with the Similax species of sarsaparilla, which has similar qualities, although apparently stronger. The wild sarsaparilla root is also a good survival food, the root providing nourishment in emergency situations.

We notice a clump of sweet fern growing adjacent to the sarsaparilla. The sweet fern isn't a true fern, as it is characterized by a woody stem, although its leaves are very fern-like in appearance. The Mi'kmaq used this plant to treat poison ivy rash. The leaves and bark were probably steeped or boiled in warm water and the liquid applied to the rash. As well, it was used in poultice form to treat rheumatism or external sores. The leaves, either green or dried, make a pleasant-tasting tea. For this purpose, steep one and a half tablespoons of green leaves or one tablespoon of dried leaves in a cup of water for five to ten minutes. You will want to experiment for yourself, as the tea can easily become strong and bitter. Lemon or honey may be added to the tea to enhance its flavour. This is a good tea to prepare while camping, or during a hike.

Lambkill, a poisonous plant, and one of the most commonly occurring and geographically widespread species in the Maritime provinces of Canada, was used as a medicinal by the Mi'kmaq. It was used to reduce swellings, and to treat rheumatic pain and sore legs and feet. The lambkill bushes were boiled in water and the liquid used as a bathing solution. A second method of treatment was to rub freshly picked leaves on the affected areas of the body.

As we move further along the gully, we find teaberry plants growing in abundance as the primary ground cover. This plant, a member of the wintergreen family and a well-known traditional medicine in both Europe and North America, is still widely recognized for its medicinal value in certain Native cultures. In the past, the Mi'kmaq used it as a blood thinner, giving it to persons who had suffered stroke or heart attack due to blood-clotting problems. The entire plant was steeped in water and taken as a tea. Another effective way to prepare teaberry medicine is to partly fill a jar with the leaves (perhaps one quarter to half full), top it with boiling water, cover, and leave it to sit in the sun or a warm place for a day or two. The result is a brew much stronger than that derived through the steeping process. The strength can be controlled by diluting the brew, or by lessening or increasing the quantity of leaves used. Use caution: prepared in this fashion, teaberry may be quite potent, especially if allowed to stand for several days. In fact, a tablespoon is probably a sufficient dosage, taken two to three times daily.

We leave that place, moving slowly through thick bushes or over areas of exposed slate towards the lake. Reaching the shore, we notice fresh deer tracks in the soft mud near the water. No doubt we alarmed the deer, who may have been munching on wild sarsaparilla stalks or some other tasty treat. We finally reach a shallow cove alive with water lilies and several species of lake grass. I mention that the Native people of the Maritimes used the root of the water lily to treat swollen limbs. The root was pounded to a pulp and applied in poultice form, or steeped in water and the liquid used as a bathing solution. The root is edible and may have been used as flour. The cow lily had similar uses.

Looking inland, Margaret notices a clump of witch hazel

growing about 20 metres from the shore. Witch hazel is an attractive small tree with a rich medicinal history, wherever it grows. For instance, it has probably been used for centuries by North American Native peoples, for both internal and external purposes. Whenever I give field walks where witch hazel is found, there are usually several people who are infatuated with the tree. This interest is due partly, of course, to the popularity of store-bought extracts of witch hazel water, and to its long, illustrious usage. People are delighted to see the actual tree growing in the wild, and to learn how to identify it; it is much like finally putting a face to the name of a person you've admired from afar for years.

Aside from the usual application of witch hazel water to external skin problems, the twigs are reputed to be an aphrodisiac. For this purpose, steep the twigs in hot water and inhale the aroma. The same procedure is considered effective in treating headache. In a pinch, simply crush the leaves in your hands and breath in their fragrance. I've often wondered if witch hazel would be useful for migraines. To prepare witch hazel tea, simply steep several leaves in a cup of boiling water for five to ten minutes, adding honey or a few drops of lemon if you wish.

III

WHILE a medicine walk is very group oriented, it is also a private, individual affair, in that each person benefits in his or her own way, and interprets the nature experience from a unique cultural and educational perspective. On this particular medicine walk, participants are encouraged to go off on their own to explore the Leipsigaek Lake area. This gives them the opportunity to experience this place privately; later on we meet near the witch hazel trees, where we form a circle to give people the opportunity to share personal experiences with the group. Frank, a veterinarian, remarks that he walked north along the lakeshore to a point of land. Resting there, he noticed an animal swimming towards the shore which, as it approached, he recognized as a muskrat. When the muskrat came ashore, it moved with remarkable quickness over the rocks, disappearing into the undergrowth. The experience convinces Frank to spend more time observing animals and bird life.

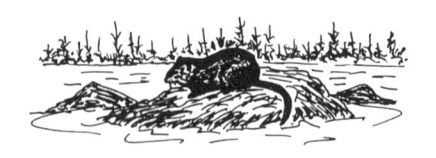

Rebecca, a music teacher, tells us she walked inland until she came to a huge boulder, which she climbed in order to relax there, observing the sights and sounds. After a few minutes she closed her eyes to meditate, but soon became restless, partly because she felt uneasy. At first Rebecca thought it was her imagination, and was determined to remain calm, with eyes closed. The feeling persisted. Opening her eyes, she noticed nothing unusual, until glancing at a group of poplar trees, she saw a hooded owl gazing directly at her. "The owl gazed at me ... it was spooky! I wasn't scared ... but I hadn't realized that an animal or a bird could do that ... it looked into my soul. I will never forget the experience." We discuss the role that owls play in folklore, legends, myths, and belief systems of traditional peoples. In some cultures, it is a bad omen for an owl to fly towards rather than away from you.

As we prepare to leave this place, I suggest that while studying plant books is valuable, and learning to recognize plants from illustrations and photographs is important, nothing can equal the value of going into the field to experience the flora first-hand. I disclose that several years earlier, while giving a plant medicine seminar, I had an experience that convinced me of the truth of this statement. I was very uptight and nervous about the seminar. To make matters worse, it was the first day-long seminar I had ever given. My tension increased when I discovered that one of the participants was a professional botanist from a New York university. I felt intimidated by his presence, but endeavoured to forget about his professional credentials, or at least to put them in the back of my mind. Yet I kept thinking, "What can I say to this guy that he doesn't already know?"

As things turned out, the seminar went very well, with the botanist making a valuable contribution to the event. He thoroughly enjoyed the plant walk, remarking afterwards how wonderful it was to see several of the plants for the first time in his life. I was speechless at his kind compliments. I was astonished that this person had studied plants for many years, but had done very little work in the field. Most of his knowledge came from the pages of books. The experience convinced me of the value of going into the landscape to learn about plants in their natural setting. I was reminded of a statement by Euell Gibbons:

> *Meditating on the first specimen of a plant*
> *that is new to me opens my eyes and sharpens my*
> *awareness until other plants of the same species*
> *become visible, standing out from the green*
> *background in an abundance that was always there,*
> *but which I was unprepared to see until I gazed*
> *deeply at a single specimen.* (p. 5)

The shoreline of Leipsigaek is very rocky, and there are areas of swamp and thick bushes, making walking difficult. We are moving through one such area when we notice that the rocks and ground surface are covered with cranberry stalks. They are everywhere. Examining them more closely, we exchange notes on cranberry recipes—including sauces—and discuss the medicinal benefits of the berries, which, steeped in water, make an excellent tonic. They are highly astringent and are used in folk medicine for urinary tract infection and general bladder complaints.

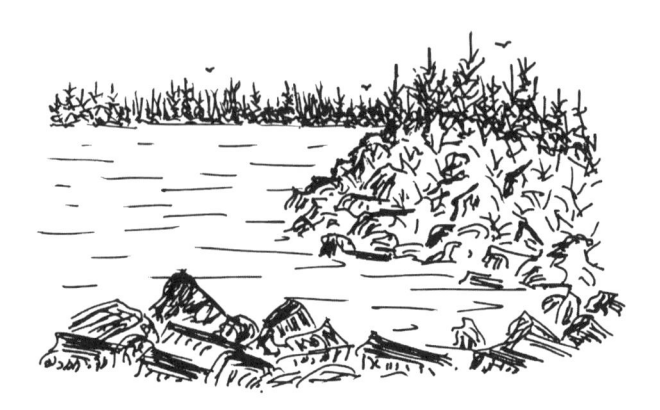

We come upon a large grove of poplar trees, growing on higher ground away from the lakeshore. Poplars were well-known and respected medicine trees in some traditional cultures. The Mi'kmaq steeped the inner bark in water as a preventative medicinal drink against colds and influenza. It was also considered effective in treating worms in humans and other animals. The bark may be baked and broken down into a powder, and used as a tea. When treating animals, the powder may have been mixed with food. There are many other important uses for Populus species, including the treatment of urinary infection and vaginal and prostate problems. Many of these remedies have never been tested by modern scientific methods, yet have been used for centuries in folk medicine.

Following the shore, we proceed across a series of flat bedrock formations to the back of a cove, where a solitary hawthorn bush grows amongst bayberry and huckleberry plants. It is surprising and delightful to find a hawthorn in this area. We are not able to identify which species of hawthorn it is, as a number of varieties can be difficult to distinguish. In fact, Roland and Smith write that over one thousand species have been noted to grow in the eastern part of North America (p. 439). Maud Grieve indicates that in Europe, Hawthorn has long been known to have cardiac, diuretic, astringent, and tonic properties (p. 385). The flowers and berries are both used, and in some instances, the leaves are also used in medicinal preparations. Terry Willard remarks that hawthorn often has to be used over long periods for its effects to be realized (p. 110). The Native peoples of North America were generally very aware of the medicinal properties of hawthorn. For instance, the Blackfoot people have used the dried berries as a mild laxative (Hellson, p. 66).

I lead the group inland, away from the lake. We have walked for perhaps 50 yards when, approaching a small swampy area, we see several large patches of labrador tea. This plant is indigenous to much of eastern Canada, and must have been used by Native peoples for centuries. The leaves were smoked as a tobacco substitute, steeped in water for tea, or used for general tonic purposes. More specifically, the tea was used to treat kidney ailments such as kidney stones. Some people confuse labrador tea with lambkill. However, it can be identified with certainty by noting the fuzzy undersides of its leaves, whose edges curl under.

We proceed slowly through barren, rocky terrain, past

the remains of half-rotten trees, parched white by years of sun and weather, until we come to an old mining road, with a grassy area where a small dwelling once stood, its foundation still evident. We find a number of medicinal plants growing here, including the mullein, flourishing in the light, sandy, rocky soil. The leaves of the mullein have a long history of usage as a treatment for asthma. The Mi'kmaq smoked them, tobacco fashion, inhaling the smoke to clear their lungs. The leaves were also steeped in water; their fumes inhaled to relieve the breathing difficulties associated with asthma. The tea must be strained well, or the small hairs from the leaves will irritate the throat. The general dosage is usually about one ounce of leaves to a pint of water, steeped for ten minutes, and taken in wine-glass quantities several times daily.

Common plantain was introduced to North America from Europe, although some botanists have concluded that it is partly native (see Zinck, vol. 2, p. 713). In fact, when I asked the Mi'kmaq about plantain, many of the elders referred to it as "white man's plantain," because "it seems to follow in the white man's footsteps. Wherever he settles, the plantain grows." These people felt strongly about the medicinal benefits of plantain. The leaves were used in poultice form to heal wounds and sores, or taken internally to treat stomach ulcers. To prepare the plant for internal use, one ounce of the leaves or seeds is steeped for ten minutes in a pint of water; one cup of the tea is taken two or three times daily.

Wild strawberry leaves are also useful in treating stomach pain and cramps. I have tried them for this purpose and found the remedy excellent. They may also be used to treat dysentery and weak intestines. The leaves should be steeped in water, or simply chewed. A general dosage is six teaspoons of fresh or dried leaves to a pint of boiling water, steeped 15 minutes. One cup of tea is taken twice daily.

Near the edge of the grassy area is a tall bull thistle. It has rather large, strikingly beautiful thistles. There are many uses for thistle species. When peeled, the central stem is edible as a wild food, as are the young flower buds. The leaves infused in water make a folk-medicine diuretic and tonic. As well, the root is astringent, and has been used to treat dysentery and diarrhea.

IV

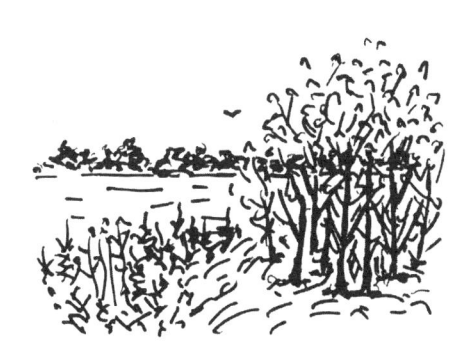

It is late afternoon as we walk the mine's road back to our point of departure. The medicine walk has taken us in a large circle within the Leipsigaek gold fields. Some members of the group are tired and anxious to go home, while others lag behind, chatting among themselves. A few people, however, have maintained the focused, meditative attitude they had at the beginning of our walk. Passing a grove of beech trees, I am reminded of the story my father told me about when he had tuberculosis in the early 1950s. A Mi'kmaq woman suggested he treat it with "winter beech" leaves. "Winter beech" refers to the dry beech leaves that remain on the trees during the winter months. She told my father to steep several leaves in a cup of water, and to drink the tea for his TB or lung problems. This tea may have been an important Native medicine during the late nineteenth and early twentieth centuries, as people were groping for ways to treat that terrible affliction. The bark and leaves of beech have strong antiseptic qualities, helpful in the prevention of infections. For example, one can wash wounds with a strong decoction of the leaves or inner bark. This is especially useful in emergency situations, where ointments and other anti-infection applications aren't available. For such external purposes, the leaves or bark may be steeped or boiled for several minutes. Beech tea was used as a general tonic, or to treat intestinal infections. The tea is made with one ounce of leaves steeped for 10 to 15 minutes in one and a half pints of water; two cups are taken daily.

Continuing on our walk, we notice burdock and red clover plants growing in a ditch along the mining road. Burdock is a wonderful medicine for skin ailments such as rashes, itching, or other irritations. The roots were steeped in water and taken as a tea to purify the blood. It is made with one ounce of the dried root to one and a half pints of water, steeped for 15 minutes. The average dose is two to three cups daily.

Red clover is also excellent for the blood, and a good companion to burdock for blood tonic purposes. Like burdock, it is useful for skin problems caused by impurities in the blood. As well, the Mi'kmaq used red clover tea to treat feverish conditions. It is made with one ounce of the dried plant to one pint of water, steeped for ten minutes. One or two cups of the tea are taken daily for tonic purposes. There are many other medicinal uses for the red clover plant. Some herbalists use it to stimulate the liver and gall bladder, to relieve constipation, and as a gargle for sore mouth and throat.

Finally arriving back at our point of departure, I finish the medicine walk by discussing briefly the rules and guidelines for collecting plants. I note that there are several general rules to keep in mind while collecting wild plants for medicines or teas. For example, the size and shape of plants and roots are often determined by growing conditions, and by the overall environment in which the plant is located. It is usually wise to look for plants or roots with a hardy character. The theory behind this is that plants that struggle to survive are better medicinally, because the struggle has strengthened them. They are said to have "strong personality." Other plants of the same species may have favourable growing conditions, making them large and healthy looking, but they may not be as potent. Of course, this is not to suggest that you ignore large, healthy-looking plants, as they are quite likely to be medicinally effective. However, it does suggest that simply because a plant is large, or has the best growing conditions, this does not necessarily make it the best medicine. Personally, I like this approach to collecting and studying plants, as it includes a consideration of the plant's environment and life experiences. Plant collecting is a learning process and, in the end, experience will become your best guide. Through practice, the taste, texture, shape, and growing conditions of a root will all be important in the collecting of plants for medicines and teas.

The weather is another important consideration, as one should try to collect under the most favourable conditions: dry, sunny weather is excellent for this purpose. Generally speaking, the medicinal potency of plants is reduced by rain, or by allowing plants to soak in water. Wet plants are more likely to spoil, which is another reason not to collect under these conditions. Also, plants probably retain more of their oily substances under dry conditions.

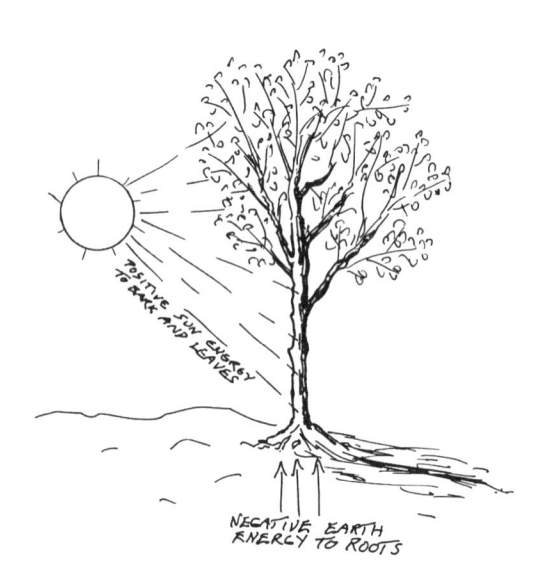

From a Native perspective, the most favourable period to collect plants is from sunrise (when the sun first casts its positive life energy on the plants) to early afternoon, or certainly before the sun begins to decline. During this period there is a favourable balance between the earth's energy, which the plant or tree is receiving through its root system, and the sun's energy, which the plant absorbs through its leaves and other exposed areas. If you are collecting bark from trees, it is essential to collect from the side of the tree on which the sun is shining. Avoid the dark side. This maximizes the positive life energy from the sun, and ritually indicates that you are in balance with light and life. To avoid damaging a tree, it is important to remove bark in small amounts or from side branches.

Location is yet another consideration when collecting plants. High locations are good, where the soil is dry and the air is fresh. Of course, much depends on the plant species you are collecting; certain plants are only found in low, wet areas. Do not collect plants along the roadside if you intend to apply them on your body or internally. It is a good idea to allow a distance of 40-70 feet between yourself and the road when gathering plants, particularly on frequently travelled roads (Willard, pp. 16–17).

V

PARTING to go our respective ways, I know that this medicine walk has been a refreshing, even moving, experience for many of us. We have had private moments, yet there was also much sharing of lessons learned and new things discovered. I sense that for a few people it was the beginning of a personal transformation. For others, it was just one more step in personal journeys that started years ago. For myself, the walk reaffirmed my connection to the natural world, with its many life forms—the plants and trees and their medicines. This reaffirmation happens again and again as the years pass by. It is a personal medicine passage—a journey with no end.

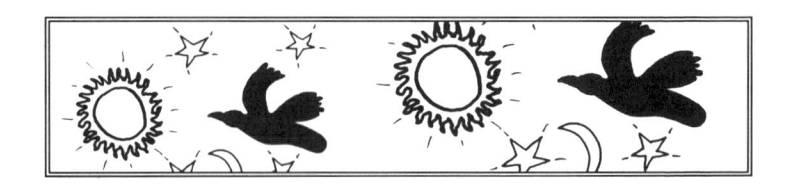

Chapter 9

THE SPIRITUALITY OF PLANTS

> *I continued to look at the flowers, and in their living light I seemed to detect the qualitative equivalent of breathing ... with no recurrent ebbs but only a repeated flow from beauty to heightened beauty....*
>
> Aldous Huxley,
> *The Doors of Perception*, p. 18

EVERY plant enthusiast has experienced the excitement and satisfaction of identifying a plant for the first time. When I began studying plant life, I was determined to gain familiarity with as many plants as possible, as quickly as I could. Whenever a Mi'kmaq person would point out or discuss particular medicine plants, I had to know how to identify them. The circumstances surrounding my research at that time forced me to delve rather quickly into the subject.

I began my plant medicine research in 1974. I remember that first summer very well because it was such a wonderful part of my life. My brother Garry and I would go into the forest and fields with our manual to identify various plants. It often took us hours to identify one, but what excitement when it happened!

> *When I finally discover a long-sought plant,*
> *I always experience a thrill of pleasure....*
> *I understand the feelings of ... medicine men*
> *who, when seeking medicinal herbs, would not*
> *pluck the first specimen found, but would sit*
> *down by it, bury a little tobacco by its roots*
> *as a thank offering, then meditate awhile, and*
> *go on until they found other plants of the same*
> *species to collect and use.*
> (Gibbons, p. 5)

The pleasure of learning to identify plants, of locating a particular plant that you have searched long and hard for, is a very satisfying and emotional high. In fact, it is spiritually nourishing, feeding and gratifying those parts of our being that are touched in the emotional and aesthetic sense. It feels good. The search itself is very therapeutic, in addition to the medicinal benefits of the plant's chemical nature. The benefits of such discovery and enjoyment have wide applications in the health field. For example, the gaining of familiarity with wild flora is a good exercise for physically and mentally challenged individuals. One way to initiate such exercise is to pair individuals or small groups with persons experienced in the identification of plant species. Also, with proper skills and experience, a recreational counsellor or therapist can lead a wild-food-foraging field trip. If the resources are available, this work can be combined with a program that teaches individuals how to grow, collect, dry, and store plants.

A second approach to wild-plant therapy is to initiate a long-term project whereby species are mapped over a given area, and growing conditions noted. A great deal of satisfaction and confidence can be gained in this undertaking. This is excellent therapy for individuals in drug and alcohol rehabilitation programs, or for those suffering from depression or low self-esteem. Working with plant life, either wild or domestic, can give a sense of meaning and spiritual well-being to one's life.

Founding a nature group or club is an excellent way to ensure that people receive the benefits of outdoor activities. Individuals can meet to exchange ideas and experiences, and to participate in group outings, such as a photography excursion. In this venture, members might photograph wild plants and catalogue the photos, perhaps donating the catalogues to schools, libraries, or university botanical departments. Think of the wonderful sense of accomplishment gained from such a program!

There are obvious situations in which a counsellor could skilfully incorporate a fine arts program with outdoor activity involving plants and nature. Under the right circumstances, it can be very relaxing to sketch and paint in an outdoor environment. The end result of such activity might be a group exhibit of paintings, drawings, and photography. Whether you are a therapist working with mentally or physically challenged individuals, or with people in drug and alcohol rehabilitation programs, plant life and the natural landscape can be of much benefit.

Of course, everything I have said in relation to group therapy can be applied on an individual basis with similar results. Anyone who reads this book can benefit greatly by experiencing the natural world more fully, and incorporating this world into their daily or weekly schedule, through painting, sketching, photography, hiking, or simply studying the great variety of plant life.

The Next Step: The Spiritual Lessons of Plants

In earlier chapters we explored the use of plants and trees as medicines and foods. Now it is time to take another step in our exploration—to examine the use of plants in relation to creative visualization, meditation, and spirituality. I am inspired by the knowledge that many traditional cultures consider plants to be sacred life forms. In these cultures, plants have special powers and are believed to be under the protection of psychic and spiritual forces or entities. I believe this far-reaching concept of plant life has great potential if applied within broad therapeutic models in modern Western culture, and that plants may be used successfully to promote the overall health and well-being of people in our fast-paced technological society.

This approach requires people to move beyond their present understanding or world view to entertain alternate views of reality. This alone, if undertaken willingly, has a positive effect on the creative imagination, in that it challenges us to be flexible—to stretch our minds, so to speak—and to consider things we have not imagined before. To consider the spiritual world of plants requires humility, the same humility required of a novice about to embark on a wonderful learning adventure—perhaps the study of sculpture or painting from a master artist. Furthermore, to learn the spiritual lessons of the plant world requires a person to observe and learn with the totality of their being. They should be sensitive to impressions received through the inner faculties as well as the faculties of the objective mind.

Legends play a key role in the teaching and learning processes in traditional societies. Unfortunately, due to rapid cultural change and the spread of modern Western ideas, ideals, and physical culture, many traditions and legends are lost. To some extent, traditional plant knowledge remains strong in certain areas of the rain forests of South America; although even there, changes are taking place at such a rapid rate that many cultures and their ancient knowledge are in danger of disappearing, or have already disappeared from the face of the earth.

Mark Plotkin, ethnobotanist, documents the rich healing traditions of the rain forest tribes. He writes about certain potent medicinal and ceremonial plants that probably find a place in the oral legends and myths of the people using them. Plotkin describes *epena*, a legendary hallucinogenic plant substance taken by the Yanomamo to summon the hekura, or little men of the jungle—spirit beings who help the shaman cure diseases and perform magic feats. Participating in an epena ceremony, Plotkin writes, "The little figures at the edge of my field of vision multiplied in number as they danced faster and faster.... I asked the shaman who the little men were.... 'They are the hekura,' he replied, 'the spirits of the forest'" (p. 266).

Peyote, of course, is one of the better-known legendary ceremonial plants. It is considered very sacred in Navajo culture, for instance, and is at the centre of ceremonies performed by the Native American Church. Jonathan Ott remarks that peyote was a ritual hallucinogen in ancient Aztec culture. They called it peyotl, which means "furry thing," an allusion to the tufts of hairs crowning mature plants (p. 48). Today it probably finds use in Tarahumara, Huichol, and Cora cultures of northern Mexico, among others. Aldous Huxley's *The Doors of Perception* spurred interest in the plant in modern western culture. This interest peaked with the 1969 release of Carlos Castaneda's *The Teachings of Don Juan: A Yaqui Way of Knowledge*.

The eastern woodlands peoples, including the Mi'kmaq of Atlantic Canada, must have had a rich legend tradition concerning the spiritual and ceremonial nature and purposes of plants. While much of this knowledge is lost, largely due to early and sustained contact with Europeans, some of it survived. For example, much of the teaching and traditions associated with sweet grass must be very old.

In the 1890s, an American folklorist, Stansbury Hagar, came to Nova Scotia to research Mi'kmaq culture. He visited the Digby area, and in 1896, published "Micmac Magic and Medicine," in the *Journal of American Folk-Lore*, based on material collected during his sojourn in Nova Scotia. This is one of the few written accounts that give us an inkling of Mi'kmaq plant legends. The material in his account is tantalizing, and makes us long for more. I wish I had been around in the 1890s when Hagar was doing his research. There is something very interesting about the man, and, from a folklore perspective, his work is important, because he gives us a glimpse into Mi'kmaq culture that is otherwise unavailable.

Hagar writes of a plant the Mi'kmaq called *mededeskooi*, the "rattling plant." The plant has three leaves that strike together with the sound of the rattlesnake. It stands about knee-high, with leaves eight inches long, shaped like those of the poplar. The root is the size of a man's fist, and the stalk is surrounded with numerous brownish-yellow balls the size of buckshot. The Mi'kmaq with whom Hagar spoke described the plant as resembling the wild turnip. They probably meant the segabun, or

Indian turnip. This is the plant I thought about when I first read the description.

Hagar writes that he met only one person who claimed to have seen the plant, and that generally the Mi'kmaq were reluctant to talk about the *mededeskooi*. Stephen Bartlett, who claimed to have seen it, described the plant as smaller than he had expected. When he returned the following morning, the plant had disappeared. Apparently, this was because he had neglected to perform the proper ceremony, or to approach the plant in the correct manner. The reference to the plant disappearing says something about the otherworldly or spiritual nature of plants in Mi'kmaq culture. There are two possible interpretations: either the Mi'kmaq considered these plants to be a special class of spiritual plant life compared with ordinary plants growing in the wild, or they felt that certain plants in the landscape (for example, the Indian turnip) possessed the ability to disappear or change location. Whatever the case, the account illustrates a view of plant life and living things that is foreign to modern botany, science in general, and Western thought.

Hagar also writes that you must follow the *cooasoonech* (a bird dwelling in old logs), who will take you to the plant, which will otherwise remain invisible. When the bird sings, follow it until eventually you hear the rattling leaves of the magic plant. Shortly afterwards the plant will appear. Then you must gather 30 sticks and lay them in a pile near the plant, before leaving that place. When you return, it must be with a girl—the more beautiful the better—and both of you must approach the plant crawling on hands and knees. The plant is inhabited by the spirit of a rattlesnake, which will come forth and circle the plant. You must pick up the snake, which will then disappear. Hagar completes his description:

> The plant must be divided into four portions ... three may be taken ... one must be left standing. The three parts are scraped and steeped and a portion wore about the person. Some say that, divided in seven parts, this medicine will cure seven diseases, but the great majority believe that it will cure any disease and gratify any wish. It is held to be especially potent as a love-compeller. (pp. 176-77)

The reference to the rattlesnake is interesting, in light of the fact that it does not live in the eastern part of the continent. Also, Hagar's comment that the medicine can be worn "about the person" to prevent illness, is characteristic of several other Mi'kmaq medicine plants, including the flagroot (sweet flag), *segabun* (Indian turnip), and *pagosi* or *bugosi* (cow parsnip).

Wilson and Ruth Wallis, in their ethnography of the Mi'kmaq, mention a plant similar in some respects to the *mededeskooi*:

> *Another good medicine ... is a tall plant which has six leaves, in pairs, one pair directly over the other. Some men who found it blazed a tree alongside it, so that they could find it later. When they returned to get it they ... could not find it. I myself, in company with some others, found one. We left our axes by it, and went to dinner. When we returned ... it was gone. An old woman once told me, "you must put a penny on the ground, over the roots; the plant will then not go away." In the old days people placed the kneecap of an animal over its roots, and the plant would then not go away. If you drink tea made from it and rub some of the plant on your hands and face, you can sleep next to a person with smallpox or anything else, and you will not contact the disease.* (p. 129)

The comment that the plant "was gone" may indicate the power of movement on the part of the plant, or refer to its ability to become invisible or a pure spirit essence. The idea of a plant moving back and forth between a physical manifestation and an invisible spirit world may not have been considered unusual, since in Native cultures there generally isn't a sharp distinction between the physical and spiritual realities; indeed, they are viewed as a single continuum of life. This is one reason why spiritual healing is considered effective.

II

THE Mi'kmaq considered certain plant compounds to be potent medicines; so potent, in fact, that they took on legendary importance. Stansbury Hagar discusses a special compound medicine made from seven ingredients: alum bark, hornbeam bark, beech bark, wild willow bark, wild blackberry bark, ground hemlock root, and red spruce root. They must be gathered in autumn and in the order given. He also describes how to collect the barks and roots, and mentions that the compound is used for both internal and external purposes:

> *The trunk of every tree is divided into four sections supposed to face the sun between sunrise, at dawn, noon, sunset, and midnight. In the forenoon one should cut the bark from the direction of sunrise as far as the direction of the sun at noon, but no further. This is the most propitious quarter, hence medicine gathered from it will yield the best results. In the afternoon cut from the noon point to the sunset point. This quarter is propitious, though less so. Bark gathered from the*

other two quarters or from the right quarter at the wrong time is at least useless, often poisonous. For the sunlight purifies the side it touches, but the shadow is hostile to life. The roots should extend from the trunk towards the propitious side. (p. 174)

These comments support the notion that it was important to collect and prepare medicines in the correct manner; otherwise they were ineffective or even poisonous. It is reasonable to assume that in traditional Mi'kmaq society, such knowledge was passed on through an apprentice system, and that it likely took years to fully learn and practise all of the medicine traditions.

In Conne River, Newfoundland, I met a person who was familiar with the collection and preparation of a compound medicine similar to the one Hagar mentions. It is called the "Seven Sorts" medicine, and at that time, was considered a panacea by a number of elderly residents. Many were familiar with the general use of this medicinal compound, and there were numerous stories of its healing powers. Yet it seemed to me that few people knew the compound's actual contents, or how to prepare it. Those who did, remarked that certain of the ingredients may vary, while others remain constant. The final nature of the medicine depends somewhat on who prepares it.

One variation of this compound medicine is made from equal amounts of the inner bark of poplar, hackmatack, dogwood, bird or pin cherry, pussy willow, and ground juniper. Black cherry bark may be substituted for the pin cherry bark. These ingredients are combined with a proportion of gold thread approximately equal in strength to each of the other ingredients. The mixture is then steeped or boiled in water depending on whether it is to be used for internal or external purposes. For internal use, the bark is steeped and the liquid taken in beverage form. For external use, the mixture is boiled until a black, molasses-like state is achieved. The medicine is applied in poultice form to the injured area.

The Seven Sorts compound is used to treat most ailments. When applied as a poultice it will help to mend broken bones, treat bruises, relieve a sore back, and heal skin cancer. The curative process followed by the compound is legendary to the people of Conne River. Tradition states that the poultice or plaster will move during the healing process. I was informed that during the course of treatment, the pain—of a back ailment, for example—will tend to move from the body in a downward direction. It is said that a Seven Sorts poultice will move in the direction the pain takes as it leaves the body. When the pain disappears, and a cure is effected, the poultice will fall from the body.

During a visit to Eskasoni, I discovered that the pussy willow, in poultice form, is said to move over the body in a manner similar to the Seven Sorts medicine. It too should be boiled to a dark molasses-like state, and is considered useful in treating most ailments. Although the Mi'kmaq I contacted in Eskasoni were unfamiliar with the Seven Sorts compound, the instructions for preparing pussy willow medicine, and its uses, were identical to those described for the Seven Sorts.

While the ingredients comprising the Seven Sorts medicine are different from those listed by Hagar for his compound preparation, there may be a relationship. I believe the Mi'kmaq were aware of the Seven Sorts preparation, even in Hagar's day. For example, Hagar remarks that "the most powerful of all known in Micmac

Pussy willow

materia medica [is] ... a mixture of seven such compounds as the one just described. It therefore contains forty-nine ingredients." It is possible that the Seven Sorts medicine is one of those seven compounds, or a variation thereof.

In this short review, I have tried to show how traditional cultures as diverse as those of the rain forests of South America, northern Mexico, the southwestern United States, and Atlantic Canada, all acknowledge the spiritual dimension of plants. Traditions vary greatly, of course, but a common thread is the belief that plants have a spiritual life, and in many instances, that plants are the windows through which humans may experience that psychic/spiritual world. I believe we may step through those windows and cross that threshold, with plants as our allies.

Plants and Dreams

Dreaming played an important role in many ancient cultures. For instance, the traditional Senoi of Malaysia cultivated dreaming to a high degree. They viewed the dream as a creative act through which problems were overcome in daily life. Dreams were a means of confronting fears, including the fear of jungle animals, with which they had to cope on a daily basis (see Corriere and Hart, p. 32). On the other hand, in Maricopa and Paviotso society, for instance, dreams are a common source of illness. The children can become ill if their parents experience bad dreams (see Krippner, pp. 128–29).

In many of the First Nation's cultures in North America, songs and singing play an important role in the healing of mental and physical ailments. These songs are often first acquired and sung during vision quests, or as the result of a dream (see Garfield, p. 69). In fact, medicine people may seek healing dreams as a cure for a specific disease. A healing treatment may appear in the dream, in the form of a song or in the recognition of a specific plant, which may then be used to treat the problem.

Similarly, in Zambia, dreams can be the means by which a disease is diagnosed. The medicine person derives an accurate description of the illness through dreaming, without having to examine the patient (Krippner, p. 128). Of course, these are not ordinary dreams, as we in Western culture commonly understand them. Rather, they are probably very lucid, often self-directed, and commonly trance-induced dreams.

Psychologist Patricia Garfield uses the appearance of plants in her dreams to gage the state of her physical health. She comments that, "If my dream plants are droopy or infected, my waking condition corresponds; if they are blooming and sprouting new growth, my waking condition is likewise healthy" (p. 34). This illustrates the close relationship that may be cultivated between the dream state and waking consciousness. It also demonstrates the usefulness of dreams in a non-traditional cultural context. Garfield uses her dreams to keep abreast of her state of health. It is conceivable that with training and practice, many people could use dreams to become better informed about their physical health, personal relationships, professional careers, or even business practices. This, of course, requires a shift in how we view life, and, for most people, an enormous leap of faith away from objective, rational thought processes as the sole guiding mental force. Dreams probably represent a more instinctive, primal response to impressions than do rational thought and judgement. It is very likely that we are missing out on a valuable part of our life experience when we fail to appreciate the gift of dreaming.

Spiritual Plant Exercises

We have reached a point where we should feel free to take the leap of faith mentioned above, and to project beyond the limits of what we think is possible in life. Your success in the following exercises depends very much upon this approach. Anything less is restrictive and might limit potential results. In these exercises, we are not concerned with objective scientific parameters to the world of plant life. This would require a different approach, with strict adherence to experimental guidelines. Rather, we are exploring the emotional, intuitive side of nature and plant life, which requires the use of mind and consciousness in ways similar to those employed by a painter inspired to create a spiritually sensitive work of art, or by a composer who, in meditative and psychic reverie, is inspired to create a beautiful piece of music. We must work with the exercises as though we are artists, exploring new frontiers with our craft. Our brushes are the exercises themselves; our pigment is the spirit energy within nature; our medium is our human sensitivity; and our canvas is daily life.

A few words must be said about the theoretical orientation of the exercises. First, they are based solely on my personal meditations and observations. This is important to understand from the outset, for the following reasons. Because of the personal nature of my investigations, I cannot say with certainty that results will be the same for everyone. When I say, for example, that the lambkill plant represents "healing and the colour green," my authority is personal experience. I feel confident that most people who correctly perform the exercise will come to fully appreciate my statement. Differences may very well be the result of the diverse nature of human beings; both one's religious or spiritual orientation and state of health may influence results. Yet I am confident that most personal human differences are accommodated within the broad orientation of a plant's energies. If lambkill's energy is generally healing in nature, then it will be healing in some form to most people. This is my hypothesis.

Secondly, the spiritual plant exercises are not an attempt to emulate processes of Native shamanism or Native medicine practices. Too many people today are trying to take advantage of the popularity of traditional Native religious and spiritual practices, to make this spirituality a consumer product for the mass marketplace. Much so-called "New Age" literature falls into this category. Many of its practitioners may be referred to as "plastic" medicine men or medicine women, and are not truly trained in the traditional ways of the culture. So, if you are hoping to find traditional Native teachings on plant spirits, you might as well close this book and look elsewhere.

As noted earlier, there are ancient traditions in some areas of the world that mention spirit beings as guardians of the plants, trees, mushrooms, and other types of vegetation (see Thompkins, p. 45). These beings are referred to under many terms, even classified into different species according to appearance—e.g., fairies, brownies, elves, gnomes, nymphs, and sylphs. In India, Hindu traditions mention specific powers or spirit beings known as devis, devatas, and devas.

In the following exercises, I talk about the "spirit energy" of plants, and the ways we can benefit from this energy. I prefer this general approach, allowing each person the opportunity to form his or her own impressions concerning the spiritual nature of the world, and the role plants and trees play in it. Some people may refer to this world in terms of spiritual entities or beings; others may prefer to approach the matter in terms of energies, as I have done in this chapter. The options are open, and rest with your particular worldview and philosophical orientation.

Fir, Balsam, *Abies balsamea* (L.) Mill

There is a First Nations' legend (perhaps Mi'kmaq) associated with the fir tree, which relates that the guardian of this tree is a large spirit being whose body is covered with scabs. The scabs are oozing a powerful healing substance. These scabs with their fluid represent the balsam blisters on the trunk of the fir tree. When the blisters are punctured, the sap oozes from them and bleeds over the tree bark.

Early on in my meditations I discovered that the fir tree has an affinity for "history" and things past. By this I mean that it is proud of its legendary background; curiously, as I meditated with this tree, I found myself drawn to a consideration of history. Students who are writing history papers or reviewing for history exams would do well to study in a fir forest environment, as might others who are doing historical research or writing an historical novel.

Balsam fir

The fir tree should be approached in a respectful and dignified manner. Find an area with several mature trees. Standing among them, scatter tobacco in the four directions, beginning with the east. This is an offering to the spirit of creation and the fir species. Then, seat yourself among the trees and relax. Take three deep breaths, close your eyes, and spend several minutes focusing on the guardian spirit or special energy of the balsam fir tree. Make careful note of any impressions or images that might occur. Next, visualizing the tree itself, see its bark, twigs, and needles. Concentrate on these things, but don't strain yourself. If you notice tension in your forehead and brow area, release it, as this is a sign of strain and indicates that you are trying too hard for results.

After several minutes of concentration, release the visualization, and remain sitting. Allow impressions to flow into your mind, without interruption. You may gain fresh impressions about an event that happened earlier in your life. Or, you may receive insight into a current problem. Continue this exercise for 10 to 20 minutes. In conclusion, say a few words of thanks for the success of the exercise.

Gold Thread, *Coptis trifolia* (L.) Salisb.

The spirit energy of the gold thread will teach lessons from nature. These lessons may manifest as a series of insights during meditation or while examining the plant. This is what I have learned from the gold thread.

Locate an area where the plants are plentiful. This will usually occur in conifer or mixed forests. Give a tobacco offering to the first group of gold thread plants you find. As you make the offering, say a prayer of thanks for the opportunity to learn from this plant. Proceed to a second group of gold thread plants and sit among them. Take a plant in your fingers and examine its shape and texture in detail. Close your eyes and visualize

Gold thread

the gold thread on the screen of your consciousness. Imagine the plant as much larger than it is in physical reality. When you have a clear visualization, ask the gold thread energy to give you the gift of its teachings. Release the image and sit for several minutes, paying careful attention to whatever impressions flow into your mind. Finally, open your eyes and continue sitting, paying close attention to mental impressions and to the visual landscape itself.

Ground Pine, *Lycopodium obscurum* L. and other varieties

Locate an area where the ground pine is plentiful. If possible, seat yourself where you are surrounded by these plants. Relax. Examine the environment around you. Give an offering of tobacco to the ground pine energy and say a few words of thanks for the assistance you will receive. In this exercise, the plant will be used to increase your energy level. Calmly observe the plants. Close your eyes, visualize the plants, and concentrate on the image for several minutes. Open your eyes and again observe the environment. Examine your feelings at the moment. Note if your energy level has improved. Complete the exercise with words of thanks in your own manner.

Ground pine

Hemlock, *Tsuga canadensis* (L.) Carr.

Locate one or several tall, mature hemlock trees. Approach the hemlock with respect, because it represents great strength, power, and healing. I believe you should approach this tree when in need of strength to overcome a problem or to reach a goal. During meditation, I was impressed with the thought that when you sit with a hemlock, you are bathed in an aura of healing energy. I was also reminded that such healing energy is everywhere present in the forest. When you walk there, you are bathed in the healing properties of the trees, plants, and rocks.

Scatter tobacco in the four directions, beginning with the east. Say a short prayer to each direction as you proceed around the circle. Choose a hemlock and seat yourself near it. You can lean against the trunk of the tree if you are so inclined. Close your eyes and feel yourself flooded in the strong energy of this tree. Maintain a humble, thankful attitude and a clear mind. Be open to impressions and insight, while you continue to sit for 20 to 30 minutes. Close the exercise with words of thanks.

Horsetail, Field, *Equisetum arvense* L.

Locate a community of field horsetail plants. If possible, position yourself where you are surrounded by the plants. Relax. Casually examine the environment around you, noting the different kinds of plants, trees, and other life forms. Place a tobacco offering among the plants. Relax.

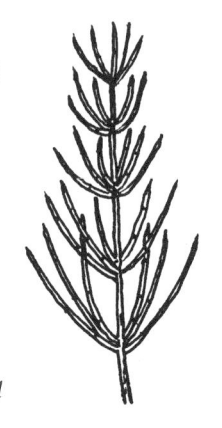

Calmly observe the plants. You may begin to feel invigorated or bathed in a field of energy. Close your eyes if you wish, and focus on this energy, or simply continue to observe the plants with open eyes. After a period of 10 to 20 minutes, close the exercise with words of thanks.

Juniper, Common, *Juniperus communis* L.

I believe this plant signifies otherworldliness in both a psychic and spiritual sense. It is therefore a very good plant to use in conjunction with meditation practices. The scent of juniper gives it this special significance. Certain scents are highly beneficial in a spiritual sense; for example, sweet grass, sage, and roses each have special significance to medicine men or women, mystics, psychics, and alchemists. The perfume of the rose changes the vibrational atmosphere of a room, making it more conducive to the practice of spiritual exercises.

To perform this exercise you should find a location with several patches of juniper plants. Make a tobacco offering to the juniper, asking for the aid of its spiritual energies during your meditation. Seat yourself comfortably amongst the juniper so that you are surrounded by them. Relax. Feel the juniper twigs with your fingers, paying attention to their texture. Rub the twigs between your fingers until they are scented with juniper perfume. Hold your fingers near your nostrils and slowly inhale the strong scent. Exhale. Repeat the process three times. On the fourth inhalation, focus on the spirit nature of the plant, rather than on its scent. Silently ask for assistance. Exhale. Repeat twice more for a total of six breaths. Remaining relaxed with eyes closed, feel yourself drifting

Common juniper

and floating upwards and away to the spirit world. Continue the exercise for a maximum of 20 minutes. Complete the exercise by bringing your consciousness back to your physical location. Feel your body, mentally and physically, with your hands. Open your eyes. Give thanks for the guidance you have received during the exercise.

Lambkill, *Kalmia augustifolia* L.

This plant involves magic, healing, and the colour green. Locate an area where lambkill is growing in a clump-like fashion. Give a tobacco offering to the plant. Assume a sitting position near the plants. Take several deep breaths and relax. Reach out with your arms and embrace the lambkill as if you were hugging a person. Close your eyes and focus your attention on the plants. Visualize the plants and feel them in your embrace. Touch the leaves and focus on the textual impressions from the plant.

After several minutes of concentrating in this manner, release your attention and remain seated with closed eyes, waiting for impressions. Perhaps you will see the colour green on the screen of your consciousness. This is a healing colour and signifies the healing energy from the plant. Continue the exercise for 10 to 30 minutes. As usual, conclude with words of thanks in your own fashion.

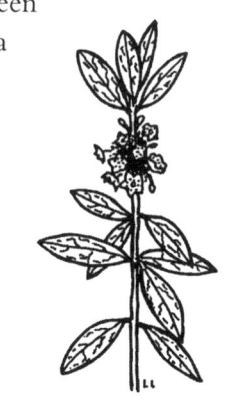

Lambkill

Mayflower (Trailing Arbutus), *Epigaea repens* L., and var. *glabrifolia*, Fern

During my meditation, I discovered that the mayflower has a calming influence on the nerves. Furthermore, the perfume of this plant is so delightful that it is emotionally beneficial to smell its blossoms regularly during spring flowering season.

Begin this exercise by giving a tobacco offering to the first group of mayflower plants you are able to locate. Ask the plant's spirit energy for assistance during the exercise. Feel the leaves of the plant with your fingers, and notice their texture. What does the pattern or design on the mayflower leaf bring to mind? After giving this some consideration, close your eyes, relax, and begin your meditation. Try to recall the wonderful scent of the flower. Feel the essence of mayflower perfume permeating the atmosphere around you and throughout your body. Relax, let go, and bathe in this essence. Allow impressions to flow into your mind. Continue this meditation for ten minutes. Afterwards, if possible, conclude the exercise by reclining in a prone position. Do whatever your body tells you to do; look up at the sky and the trees around you, or close your eyes, relax, sleep, and dream.

Mayflower

Pine, White, *Pinus Strobus* L.

In the world of trees, the pines hold a position similar to that held by the crow or raven among bird species. I'm referring largely to the expression of personality and character. Crows and ravens are very clever, expressing their intelligence in unique ways. Similarly, pine trees express uniqueness of character in the varied and unusual shapes they assume, depending on environmental conditions during the growth cycle.

Pine trees create an excellent environment for concentration and meditation. They grow tall towards the heavens, reminding us of heavenly and otherworldly things. A pine grove is very impressive to the physical eye, encouraging us to explore our spiritual nature and to seek after things of beauty and harmony. The call of the spirit is enhanced by the voice of the wind as it plays and sings through pine needles.

In this exercise, visit a pine forest when there is a breeze blowing. Give a tobacco offering to the pines. Assume a meditative posture, focusing your attention on the sound of the wind blowing through the pines. This is a good concentration exercise with benefits similar to mantra-based meditation practices. Continue the concentration for a period of 10 to 30 minutes. Then, if you feel so inclined, lie on your back and rest. You may fall asleep at this time, to experience a dream journey or to receive other impressions. Conclude your visit to the pines by giving thanks in the usual manner.

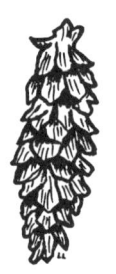

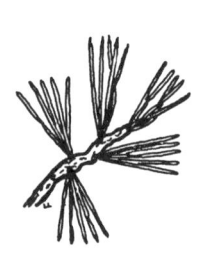

White pine

Sarsaparilla, Wild, *Aralia nudicaulis* L.

This is a very beautiful plant, particularly when growing in abundance and covering the forest floor. In these places, you may find dozens of the plants growing, all interconnected by the same root system. The wild sarsaparilla grows separate long stems for their berries. The berries attain a lovely purple colour when ripe.

Find an area where the plants are plentiful. Scatter tobacco in the four directions prior to sitting, as an offering to the spirit energy of the plant and to the spirit of creation. Seat yourself among the plants, close enough to examine the leaves of several plants with your fingers. Notice the texture of the leaves and stem. Taste a ripe berry if the opportunity presents itself. As you examine the plant, think of it as powerful medicine.

Wild sarsaparilla

For me, this plant exerts a calming influence and a feeling of peace. You may notice similar qualities. Continue to observe the plants for approximately ten minutes; closing your eyes, remain sitting another five minutes, taking note of your feelings. Conclude the exercise with words of thanks.

Spruce, Black, *Picea mariana* (Mill.) BSP

The black spruce is found in or near swamps and bogs, or in rocky terrain along the shores of lakes or near the ocean. In my meditations I learned that this tree represents purification, which will be the focus of this exercise.

Proceed to an area where several black spruce are growing. Stand in the general vicinity of the trees and make a

Black spruce

tobacco offering to the four directions, giving thanks to the spirit in your heart and to the spirit energy of the black spruce for direction during the exercise. Approach one of the trees, examining its bark and feeling the rough texture with your hands. Assume a sitting position near the tree and think about the bark, attempting to recall its textural sensations and appearance. When you have clear impressions of these things, ask the black spruce spirit for purification. Relax, feel this purification taking place—notice the impressions that enter your mind at this time. Continue the exercise for approximately 20 minutes.

Spruce, Red, *Picea rubens* Sarg.

This tree is abundant throughout much of North America. If you live where the red spruce grows, you should have little difficulty locating a suitable environment for this exercise.

Part One:

Begin with a tobacco offering to the directions, giving thanks in the usual manner for guidance received during this period. Assume a sitting position among the trees and relax. Take several deep breaths. Concentrate on the concepts of spirit energy, nature spirits, or guardian angels. How do you react emotionally and intellectually to those concepts? Realize that there will be many answers to this question, rather than a single correct answer. The main point is to answer the question honestly, and to realize where you stand in relation to these spiritual concepts, since your position on this matter will determine how you approach the exercises in this book and, ultimately, the value you derive from them.

Red spruce

Part Two:
Visualize the red spruce tree and ask it to help you to overcome your fears. Release the visualization and remain relaxed. Allow impressions to flow into you mind; if these impressions involve events or things that make you fearful, try to face those fears by calmly viewing the impressions as they flow through your mind. Continue this exercise for a maximum of 20 minutes.

Teaberry, *Gaultheria procumbens* L.

The teaberry can be used to reaffirm our connectedness to mother earth. This plant is short and grows close to the soil, so that when we sit and examine its leaves, we are reminded of the earth.

Begin the exercise by seating yourself in a patch of teaberry plants. Give a tobacco offering and prayer to the spirit of your heart, to mother earth, and to the spirit energy of the plant. Calmly examine the plants and note how they grow together as a community. After several minutes of this observation, close your eyes and visualize yourself eye level with the plants. Because they grow near the ground, you may feel the presence of the earth very strongly. Relax. Sustain your visualization while, at the same time, seeing and feeling the close presence of the earth. Continue the exercise for another 10 to 20 minutes.

This exercise is perhaps the most difficult. Do not be disappointed if you are unable to achieve satisfactory results at first. The exercise requires good visualization skills, with the ability to see the earth's surface with its teaberry plants while also feeling its nearness to you. With practice, you will be successful.

Teaberry

Wild Lily of the Valley, *Maianthemum canadense* Desf.

When I meditate or concentrate in the presence of this plant, I am impressed with thoughts of love, joy, and inspiration. The plant is therefore useful to persons seeking inspiration in such arts as writing, painting, and the theatre.

Approach the plant with respect and make an offering in a manner you find appropriate. Relax. Examine the texture of the plant with your fingers and note its main characteristics. Focus your attention and concentration on the plant. Ask for inspiration, love, and joy. Close your eyes, noting the impressions you receive, paying careful attention to those that pertain to your request. After 10 to 15 minutes, open your eyes and conclude the exercise with words of thanks and deep respect.

Lily of the valley

Willow, Pussy, *Salix discolor* Muhl., and other varieties

The pussy willow has a great deal of healing energy. This became evident early in my meditations. In this exercise, you should begin with a tobacco offering to the first group of pussy willow plants you locate, asking for assistance from the spirit energy of this particular willow, and requesting that the healing energy of the plant manifest itself in your life. When you have completed the offering, move to a second group of the plants, assume a comfortable position, relax, close your eyes, and gently hold several of the willow stalks in your hands.

Pussy willow

Concentrate for a few moments on the texture of the bark, mentally requesting its healing energy. Continue to hold the plants in your hands while passively observing the impressions that flow across the screen of your consciousness. After ten minutes of this meditation, open your eyes, releasing the willows from your hands. Remain seated. Take a minute to examine your present condition. Finish with words of thanks in your own fashion.

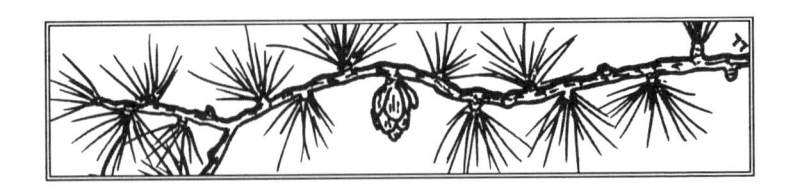

MEDICINAL PLANT/TREE INDEX
(with Preparation Instructions)

Alder, *Alnus crispa* (Ait) Pursh, and *Alnus rugosa* (DuRoi) Spreng

For external use, heat leaves in a warm oven until they curl, removing them before they become brittle. Place on sore or inflamed area of the body, keeping in place with a bandage. If the leaves later produce a burning sensation, remove and replace with a new covering of warmed leaves. For internal usage, use one tablespoon dry inner bark and/or leaves to one cup of water. Steep for ten minutes and strain. Use only occasionally (maximum one-cup dosage). Do not use alder regularly as a tonic or pleasure tea. Warning: do not take alder internally in a green state, as it may cause cramps (see pp. 80-81).

Alder

Beech, *Fagus grandifolia* Ehrh.

Use one ounce of the leaves and/or bark to one and a half pints of water. Steep for 15 minutes and strain the liquid into a container. Use occasionally as a pleasure tea or take two cups daily for medicinal purposes, for one or two weeks (see pp. 93-94).

Beech

Bull Thistle, *Cirsium vulgare* (Savi) Tenore

Use one tablespoon of leaf and/or root material to one cup of water; steep for 10 to 15 minutes. For general tonic purposes, use two cups daily for two to four weeks (see p. 93).

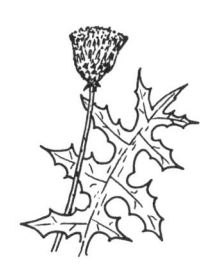

Bull thistle

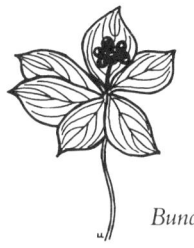

Bunchberry, *Cornus canadensis* L.

Use four to six fresh leaves, or one tablespoon crushed dried leaves, to one cup of water; steep for ten minutes (see p. 84).

Bunchberry

Burdock, *Arctium minus* (Hill) Bernh., and other varieties

Use one ounce root to slightly more than one pint water; steep for 15 minutes. The average daily dosage is two to three cups of tea. The leaves are also valuable medicinally; prepare them in the same way as the roots (see p. 94).

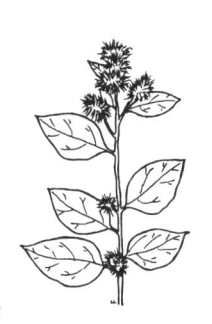

Burdock

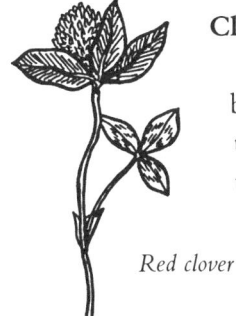

Clover, Red, *Trifolium pratense* L.

Use one ounce of the leaves and/or blossoms to one pint of water; steep for 10 to 15 minutes. The average daily dosage is two cups of tea (see p. 94).

Red clover

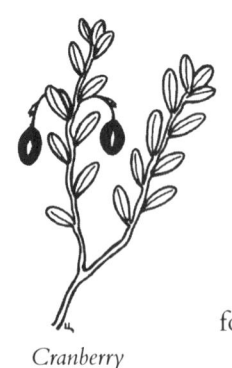

Cranberry, *Vaccinium macrocarpon* Ait.
This is an excellent tonic medicine for the urinary tract and bladder. Make the berries into a sauce, or steep a cup of berries to two pints of water for 10 or 15 minutes. Take two cups daily for seven to 10 days (see p. 90).

Cranberry

Hackmatack (Tamarack, Larch), *Larix laricina* (DuRoi) K. Koch.
Use the inner bark in a green or dried state. Use one tablespoon of bark material to one cup water; steep for 15 minutes and strain. Drink several cups of the liquid daily for colds and/or feverish conditions. For external use, the inner bark may be softened by pounding it to a pulp-like state, or by soaking it in water; apply as a poultice (see p. 82).

Hackmatack

Hawthorn, *Crataegus spp.*
The berries may be used as medicine. Use 10 to 15 drops of the fluid extract as a single dosage. Also, the flowers may be steeped in water and drank as a medicinal tea. The hawthorn is a heart tonic medicine, a diuretic, and has been used for angina as well as arteriosclerosis, among other things. It is wise to consult with a doctor and/or herbalist before taking this medicine on a regular basis (see p. 91).

Hawthorn

Labrador Tea, *Ledum groenlandicum* Oeder.

The leaves may be used dry or in a green state. Use one to two tablespoons of the leaf material to one cup water; steep for 10 to 15 minutes and drink hot or cold as a tonic. Warning: while I have yet to know of a person who has poisoned him/herself with labrador tea, care must be taken with this plant. Do not boil the leaves when preparing the tea. Boiling may release ledol, a potentially poisonous substance (see p. 91).

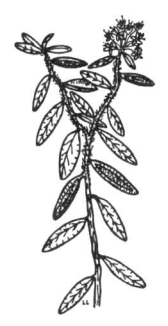

Labrador Tea

Lambkill, *Kalmia augustifolia* L.

This plant was used for external purposes by the Mi'kmaq of Atlantic Canada. The plant is poisonous and should not be taken internally. To prepare as an external bathing solution, boil the leaves or a branch of the plant in water for 10-15 minutes. Apply while hot, either by bathing with a cloth or by soaking, being careful to avoid scalding the skin (see p. 85).

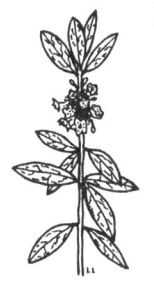

Lambkill

Lily, Cow, *Nuphar variegatum* Engelm. (*N. variegate* Durand)

The root of the cow lily is visually impressive, with its large size and scale-like texture. It reminds me of something you would expect to find in a prehistoric environment. The Mi'kmaq used the fresh root of this plant as an external poultice to reduce swellings. The root was pounded into a pulp and applied to the swollen area. It was probably held in place by a bandage or dressing of some kind. Terry Willard mentions that the Montana Indians used it to treat venereal disease, by drinking a tea from the boiled root and applying the crushed root to the affected area (see p. 87).

Cow lily

See the food plant index for more information on this valuable plant (also, see p. 86).

Lily, Water, *Nymphaea odorata* Ait.
The Mi'kmaq used this for similar purposes as the cow lily, above (see p. 86).

Water lily

Mullein, *Verbascum thapsus* L.
To prepare for internal use, steep one ounce of leaves and/or blossoms in one pint of water for 10 to 15 minutes. Strain very well, using cheese cloth, or something similar. This is an important caution, as the leaves are full of tiny hairs that may come off in the water and irritate the throat. Use one or two cups of the preparation daily (see p. 92).

Mullein

Pitcher Plant, *Sarracenia purpurea* L.
Use one teaspoon of the dried root material to half a cup of water; steep for ten minutes. Take two to three times daily, as long as required (see p. 81).

Pitcher plant

Plantain, *Plantago major* L.
Use one tablespoon of the leaf material and/or seeds to one cup of water; steep for ten minutes. Use one cup of the tea daily on a long-term basis or two to three cups daily on a short-term basis—one or two week period (see p. 92).

Plantain

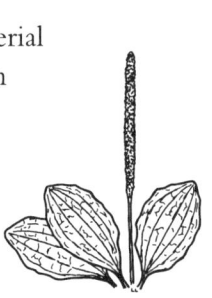

Poplar, *Populus* L. (For instance, *P. tremuloides* Michx., *P. grandidentata* Michx., and *P. alba* L.)
    The inner bark is used for internal purposes, either green or in a dry state. Use two tablespoons of the bark material to one cup of water; steep for 15 minutes. Take two to three cups of the tea daily, for a week to ten days, reducing the dose to a single cup of the tea for the following seven-day period (see p. 90).

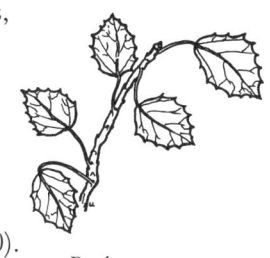

Poplar

Sarsaparilla, Wild, *Aralia nudicaulis* L.
    Use one ounce of dried root material to half a pint of water; steep for 10-15 minutes. Take two to three cups of the drink, daily (see pp. 84-85).

Wild sarsparilla

Strawberry, Wild, *Fragaria virginiana* Duchesne
    For stomach cramps, chew two to four leaves thoroughly, and swallow. To prepare as a medicinal tea, use several fresh leaves or one tablespoon of dried leaves to one cup of water; steep for 10-15 minutes. To prepare a larger amount, use six tablespoons of plant material to one pint of water (see p. 92).

Wild strawberry

Sweet Fern, *Comptonia peregrina* (L.) Coult.

Use one tablespoon of dried leaves or one and a half tablespoons of fresh leaves to one cup of water; steep for 10 minutes. This may be taken occasionally as a pleasure tea. For external use, boil the leaf and/or bark material in water for ten minutes and use as a bathing solution (see p. 85).

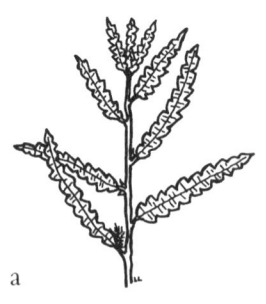

Sweet fern

Teaberry, *Gaultheria procumbens* L.

Use one and a half tablespoons of fresh leaves to a cup of water; steep for 15 minutes. Drink one to two cups daily for a maximum of two weeks. Teaberry should not be treated as an ordinary pleasure tea, because it has aspirin-like qualities and is a blood thinner. It may also be prepared by placing the leaves in a small jar until it is a quarter full. Fill the jar with boiling water, cover, and leave in a warm place for 24 hours. (Place the jar in direct sunlight, so the power of the sun can infuse the liquid. This produces a strong-smelling wintergreen liquid.) Take a tablespoon of the liquid two to three times daily for a period of two weeks (see p. 86).

Teaberry

Witch Hazel, *Hamamelis virginiana* L.

The leaves may be used in a tonic, either green or in a dry state. Use one to two tablespoons of leaf material to one cup of water; steep for 10-15 minutes. Take two cups of the tea, twice daily, for a two-week period. It also makes an interesting pleasure tea for occasional use (see p. 87).

Witch hazel

FOOD PLANT/TREE INDEX

Plant Name	Page

Arrowhead, Common, *Sagittaria latifolia* Willd. 66

Bayberry, *Myrica pensylvanica* Loisel. 67

Bearberry, *Arctosphylos Uva-ursi*, (L.) Spreng. 67

Beech, *Fagus gradifolia* Ehrh 68

Birch, Yellow, *Betula alleghaniensis* Britt. 68

Burdock, *Artium minus,* (Hill) Bernh. 69

Cattail, Broad Leaf, *Typha latifolia* L. 69
Also, *Typha angustifolia* L.

Crowberry, *Empetrum nigrum* L. 70

Dandelion, *Taraxacum officinale* Weber 71

Jewelweed, *Impatiens capensis* Meerb, ... 71
and *Impatiens pallida* Nutt.

Lettuce, Wild, *Lactuca canadensis* L., and others 72

Mountain Ash, *Sorbus americana* Marsh. 72

Nettle, Stinging, *Utica dioica* L. 73

Oak, Red, *Quercus borealis* Michx. f. and others 73

Peppermint, *Mentha piperita* L. 74

Pickerel-weed, *Pontederia cordata* L. 74

Rose, Common Wild, *Rosa virginiana* Mill., ... 75
Rosa carolina Marsh., and others

Sweet Fern, *Comptonia peregrina* (L.) Coult. 75

Sweet Gale, *Myrica gale* L. 76

Wood Sorrel, *Oxalis montana* Raf. 76

133

PLANT/TREE SPIRIT ENERGY INDEX

Plant Name	Indications	Page
Fir, Balsam *Abies balsamea* (L.) Mill	Stimulates memory, insight, and impressions from the past	113
Gold Thread *Coptis trifolia* (L.) Salisb.	Insights into nature and the natural environment	114
Ground Pine *Lycopodium obscrum*, L.	Energy tonic (increases energy levels)	115
Hemlock *Tsuga canadensis*, (L.) Carr	Healing energy bath	116
Horsetail, Field *Equisetum arvense* L.	Healing energy bath	116
Juniper, Common *Juniperus communis* L.	Otherworldliness; aid to meditation on psychic and spiritual levels	117
Lambkill *Kalmia augustifolia* L.	Magic; healing and the colour green; general healing energy	118
Mayflower *Epigaea repens* L. (var *glabrifolia* Fern.)	Calming nerve tonic	119

Plant Name	Indications	Page
Pine, White *Pinus Strobus* L.	Otherworldliness; enhances concentration and meditation practices	*120*
Sarsaparilla, Wild *Aralia nudicaulis* L.	Peacefulness and calming influences	*121*
Spruce, Black *Picea mariana* (Mill.)BSP.	Represents purification; energy purification bath	*121*
Spruce, Red *Picea rubens* Sarg.	Overcoming fears	*122*
Teaberry *Gaultheria procumbens* L.	Connectedness to Mother Earth; earth energy	*123*
Wild Lily of the Valley *Maianthemum canadense,* Desf.	Promotes impressions of love, joy and inspiration	*124*
Willow, Pussy *Salix discolor* Muhl., and other varieties	General healing energy	*124*

BIBLIOGRAPHY

Besant, Annie. *Thought Power: Its Control and Practice*. London and Benares: The Theosopical Publishing Society, 1901.

Castaneda, Carlos. *The Teachings of Don Juan: A Yaqui Way of Knowledge*. New York: Ballantine Books, 1973.

Corriere, Richard and Joseph Hart. *The Dream Makers: Discovering Your Breakthrough Dreams*. New York: Bantam Books, 1978.

Creighton, Helen. *Folklore of Lunenburg County*. Ottawa: National Museum, Bulletin 117, 1950; Toronto: McGraw-Hill Ryerson, 1975.

Elias, Thomas A., and Peter A. Dykeman. *Edible Wild Plants: A North American Field Guide*. New York: Sterling Publishing Co., 1990.

Emerson, Ralph Waldo. *Essays on Spiritual Laws and Circles*. Edited by E. Haldeman-Julius, Little Blue Book, No. 547, Girard, Kansas: Haldeman-Julius Company.

Ferguson, Marilyn. *The Aquarian Conspiracy*. Los Angeles: J.P. Tarcher Inc., 1980.

Garfield, Patricia L. *Creative Dreaming*. New York: Ballantine Books, 1982.

Gibbons, Euell. *Stalking the Healthful Herbs*. New York: David McKay Co., 1975.

Grieve, Maud. *A Modern Herbal*. Middlesex: A Peregrine Book, Penguin Books, 1976.

Hagar, Stansbury. "MicMac Magic and Medicine." *Journal of American Folklore*, Vol. 9 (1896), 170-77.

Hellson, John C. and Morgan Gadd. *Ethnobotany of the Blackfoot Indians*. Ottawa: National Museum of Man, 1974.

Huxley, Aldous. *The Doors of Perception*. New York: Harper & Row, 197

Krippner, Stanley. "Dreams and Shamanism." *Shamanism: An Expanded View of Reality*. Ed. Shirley Nicholson. Wheaton, IL: The Theosophical Publishing House, 1987. 125-132.

Krutch, Joseph Wood, Ed. *Thoreau: Walden and Other Writings*, New York: Bantam Books, 1971.

Lopez, Barry Holstun. *Desert Notes, Reflections in the Eye of a Raven*. New York: A Bard Book/published by Avon Books, 1981.

Ott, Jonathan. *Hallucinogenic Plants of North America*. Berkeley: Wingbow Press, 1976.

Plotkin, Mark J. *Tales of a Shaman's Apprentice: An Ethnobotanist Searches for New Medicines in the Amazon Rain Forest*. Toronto: Penguin Books, 1994.

Roerich, Nicholas. *Shambhala*. New York: Nicholas Roerich Museum, 1985.

Roland, A.E. and E.C. Smith. *The Flora of Nova Scotia*. Halifax: Nova Scotia Museum, 1969.

Suzuki, Shunryu. *Zen Mind, Beginner's Mind*. New York & Tokyo: Weatherhill, 1982.

Thompkins, Peter. *The Secret Life of Plants: Living in Harmony with the Hidden World of Nature Spirits from Fairies to Quarks*. New York: Harper Collins Publishers, 1997.

Wallis, Ruth and Wilson. *The Micmac Indians of Eastern Canada*. Minnesota: The University of Minnesota Press, 1955.

Willard, Terry. *Edible and Medicinal Plants of the Rocky Mountains and Neighbouring Territories*. Wild Rose College of Natural Healing, 1992.

Wilhelm, Richard, translator (translated from the German by Cary F. Baynes). *The Secret of the Golden Flower: A Chinese Book of Life*. New York: Harcourt, Brace & World, 1962.

Yogananda, Paramahansa. *Man's Eternal Quest: Self Realization Fellowship*. 1988.

Zinck, Marian, Ed. *Roland's Flora of Nova Scotia*. Halifax: Nimbus Publishing & Nova Scotia Museum, two volumes, 1998.